KEEPERS OF THE SOUL

THE FIVE GUARDIAN ELEMENTS OF ACUPUNCTURE

KEEPERS OF THE SOUL

NORA FRANGLEN

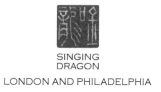

SINGING
DRAGON
LONDON AND PHILADELPHIA

Every effort has been made to trace copyright holders and to obtain their permission for the use of copyright material. The author and the publisher apologize for any omissions and would be grateful if notified of any acknowledgements that should be incorporated in future reprints or editions of this book.

This edition published in 2014
by Singing Dragon
an imprint of Jessica Kingsley Publishers
73 Collier Street
London N1 9BE, UK
and
400 Market Street, Suite 400
Philadelphia, PA 19106, USA

www.singingdragon.com

First edition published by the School of Five Element Acupuncture, 2006

Library of Congress Cataloging in Publication Data
Franglen, Nora.
 Keepers of the soul : the five guardian elements of acupuncture / Nora Franglen.
  pages cm
 Originally published: London : School of Five Element Acupuncture, 2006.
 Includes bibliographical references.
 ISBN 978-1-84819-185-3 (alk. paper)
 1. Acupuncture. 2. Mind and body. I. Title.
 RM184.F5862 2014
 615.8'92--dc23
                                            2013024594

British Library Cataloguing in Publication Data
A CIP catalogue record for this book is available from the British Library

ISBN 978 1 84819 185 3
eISBN 978 0 85701 146 6

Printed and bound in Great Britain

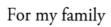

For my family

'Not a single tremor of one human being that does not affect us all.'

Charles Dickens

CONTENTS

ABOUT THE AUTHOR   9

Introduction   11

OPENING THE CIRCLE

1. The Pattern of Things   18
    The quest for our own identity   23
    The cadence of the universe   28
    The guardian of the soul   36
    The body as portrait of the soul   44
    Nature's pull towards health   51
    The elements at work   56

2. Our True Shape   61
    The guardian element   66
    Why does imbalance occur?   73
    What is balance?   79
    Has imbalance a function?   85
    Assessment of balance   90
    Sensory diagnosis   99
    Energies in process of change   106

3. Opening the Circle   114
    The elements as filters   121
    The messengers of the elements   127
    Patterns of flow   135

WITHIN THE CIRCLE

4. The Circle of the Elements   146

5. The Wood Element   151
       The signatures of Wood   157
       Wood's two officials   163
       Margaret Thatcher   167
       My Wood mother   170

6. The Fire Element   178
       The two sides of Fire   185
       Billy Connolly and Tony Blair   189
       A Fire patient   195
       Fire under pressure   198

7. The Earth Element   202
       The pull of Earth   206
       Princess Diana   211
       The elements in embryo   218

8. The Metal Element   224
       Patrick, Proust and Presley   232
       My Metal element shadow   238

9. The Water Element   241
       The shapes of Water   245
       Alex and David Beckham   251
       Our place in the circle   257

CLOSING THE CIRCLE

10. A 21st-Century Context   264
       A cry from the heart   269
       The medicalized society   276
       A vision for acupuncture   283

11. Closing the Circle   290

About the Author

Nora Franglen has a degree in Modern Languages from Cambridge University, and worked as a translator whilst bringing up a young family. Her own experience of five element acupuncture led her to study at the College of Traditional Acupuncture, Leamington Spa, UK, and she continued her postgraduate studies there under J.R. Worsley. She was Founder/Principal of the School of Five Element Acupuncture (SOFEA) in London from 1995–2007 and continues her teaching through her practice, through postgraduate work in the UK, Europe and China, and now through her blog, norafranglen.blogspot.com. She lives in London, UK.

INTRODUCTION

This present book wrote itself in the form it appears here. It had its own inner imperative and that I had to obey. I am aware that it cannot be regarded as a general introduction to acupuncture. For that, the reader must look elsewhere. It is, instead, one person's discovery of a profound truth, and reflects my need to share the awesome beauty of what I have learnt. I do not seek to persuade, for there will be many for whom what I have written appears mere fantasy and illusion, or just plain nonsense. Others may perceive some truth here, as I have felt there is, else I could not have written this.

Very little in acupuncture is familiar to a Western medical eye, and even those things that are, such as the names of the organs of the body, are deceptive in their familiarity, because they encompass other, deeper functions than the merely physical which the West recognizes. If you are new to acupuncture, you may find it easier to put aside any previous assumptions about the nature of health and ill-health, suspend your disbelief, as all good critics should, and reposition yourself at a completely different angle to the human being and human health. It is as though you are being asked to see things through a different lens. Once having shifted your focus in this way, you may find that acupuncture offers a fresh perspective on reality, which, for me, now represents a far more profound truth than the Western concepts I was brought up with.

I am writing this as a labour of love, my own homage to a discipline which has fed me personally in my own treatments, and has fed my patients as I have treated them. It still astounds me that a form of healing so uniquely appropriate for where we find ourselves now in the Western world at the start of the 21st century should be so little known about, and often, where known, so misunderstood. To clear some of the cobwebs of such misunderstandings is one of my aims, as it is to introduce this discipline to those to whom it is still a closed book. A further, somewhat different but connected aim is to help those who practise five element acupuncture gain a deeper understanding of their practice.

For many years I gave introductory evening classes on acupuncture in London. These were open to anybody and most of those attending had no previous knowledge of acupuncture at all. One of the delights for me was the ease with which each new class, made up of plumbers and secretaries and retired businessmen and young unemployed, almost without exception understood what I was talking about as being relevant to them. And this confirmed to me that I touched here upon something which I have learnt is a universal truth, for it chimed with the knowledge of human nature which all these different people brought to my classes. It has a universal resonance which at first surprised me, but which I then took so for granted that any show of sceptical disbelief, occasional though this may have been, came as a shock, as though that person in the class was blind to something all the rest of us could see. This confirmation of my conviction of the truth of what I taught and practised became a satisfactory, initially surprising, outcome of these classes, and provided the impetus for this book.

Acupuncture appears to have sprung into existence as though ready-formed. Some of its shape may well have altered with time. Things have been added to it, or taken away. It loses some of its lustre in certain epochs. It glows brightly at other times. Now we find it appearing suddenly in one country, now in another. But its light, though dimmed at intervals, never goes out, and we can trace such an unbroken line that we find it here in the West at the start of the 21st century, and already it was old when this Christian era began.

One of its beauties is that its tradition is deeply steeped in the oral, in what one practitioner has learnt and been able to pass on in his lifetime. And such a strongly oral tradition brings a freshness to it often alien to the much more rigidly formulated learning of Western sciences. I feel strongly that we must each pass on whatever knowledge we have gained so that others may make use of our years of learning and practice as we have made use of those of others before us. We owe it to what we believe in, not only to draw deeply on its traditions, but to give something back. The acupuncture school I founded was my attempt to encourage such new growth during my lifetime.

Perhaps a capacity to take things on trust must to some extent accompany any acupuncturist, for what acupuncture does, though well documented, and with much evidence to its efficacy, often fails to answer the question 'how?' I think we can fairly say that we know that it works, since countless generations of patients attest to this, but much, much more needs to be done if the 'how' is to be understood. For my part, this has never worried me, indeed has added to acupuncture's fascination for me, for its apparent use of the elusive and intangible reinforces its potential, and one made much of in this book, to affect within us the mysterious worlds of the soul. Such a powerful action needs to call for support upon forces which perhaps no measuring flask or scientific instrument can be allowed to capture. We can no more encapsulate, for example, the experience of loving another person in simple words than we can define in simple terms that coming together of the energetic interfaces of two people, the patient and his practitioner, which forms the core of an acupuncture treatment.

The action of manipulating a needle in a given acupuncture point on the skin can be described thus without difficulty: 'Locate the acupuncture point by means of specific anatomical landmarks. Place the needle on the point, and insert to a given depth. Manipulate the needle in a given way, and remove.' Nothing here to hint of anything to worry the scientific mind.

The application and the needling action are reassuringly physical. Add that extra ingredient, however, which gives to that selection of that point and that insertion of the needle a deeper significance, and the reassuring world of the physical, with its quantifiable, measurable effects gives way to something much more intangible. How can that very physical needle with its very physical action upon the physical skin make a patient angrier or sadder, light up a patient's eyes or bring a smile to a patient's lips? And all of these effects can happen after any treatment.

Where then do we turn for an explanation? The physical has evoked something which is more than a merely physical reaction. The smile is not just a physical turning up of the lips and a physical crinkling of the eyes, but an expression of some inner joy within the patient, which all of us respond to with our own emotional responses. Where is our response coming from? What is being evoked that stimulates an emotional response of this kind in us?

To this layer of response we give, among others, the word spirit. For reasons of my own I often prefer the word soul, for soul has not yet been debased, as spirit has, by its overuse in such expressions as body, mind and spirit, now fast becoming a cliché. How much of the spirit is actually found at a Body Mind and Spirit Festival, for example? The soul retains a resonance of the awesome, of that which awes us, sadly lost to spirit, and evokes an echo of that deeper world inside us, that 'something of the gods' which has drawn each one of us up out of the primaeval slime into the gleaming worlds which beckon far beyond and deep within us. These depths, both within and beyond, are immeasurable, to be kindled by such things as the reading of a poem or listening to music or a moment of beauty at sunrise or sunset.

This soul cannot be described, cannot be analyzed, cannot be fragmented into words, ineffable in the truest meaning of that word, that still centre at the heart of us beyond which we cannot venture, breathed in to the first cell to give it life, and breathed out with our last breath to bring us death. To touch, however lightly, our physical container, is to touch, however lightly, our soul. And it is about the human soul that I want to speak here, a thing of infinite beauty, yet we may crush it, sometimes voluntarily, and that is wickedness and evil, and sometimes involuntarily, and that is carelessness and often self-neglect.

A needle, I have learnt, can touch upon these depths. It can stir their numbness to life or deaden their pain. It is the manipulation of such a needle for such a purpose that is the main focus of this book.

Needle can touch Spirit

I have called the three sections of this book 'Opening the Circle', 'Within the Circle' and 'Closing the Circle' to reflect the non-linear, circular processes which underlie acupuncture. This reflects, too, the cycles of energy which flow from outside to within and through us back to the outside world.

The writing of this book has been a similar cyclical process for me, in which the thoughts with which I started changed and developed as I translated them from my own personal language into the more universal language of a book. The person who started writing this was a different person from the one who is now writing these last reflections, a further sign that in every end is another beginning. I like to think that the last words of this book will lead readers back to this introduction, adding a further loop to the spiral of their understanding.

OPENING THE CIRCLE

CHAPTER 1

THE PATTERN OF THINGS

A reader unfamiliar with acupuncture will now have to make a leap of faith until what I write here has made a sufficiently convincing argument for acupuncture, or, failing to convince, has led them to lay this book aside.

I, too, when I approached my own first acupuncture treatment many years ago, had to make a similar leap of faith to bring myself to the acupuncturist's couch. I had come to this treatment with only the vaguest knowledge of acupuncture. I can still remember how surprised I was that needles were not inserted into my ears, as I had seen on TV once, and that my acupuncturist wanted to know so much about me. Since my background was steeped in Western medicine, I had never till then doubted Western medicine's efficacy nor was I aware that there might be other ways of viewing health or treating ill-health. Looking back now, I am amazed at my almost placid acceptance of the medical status quo and at how incurious I was.

All this was shattered by the effects of my first treatment. And these effects were all the more disturbing for being so unexpected. I had gone into this treatment with little expectation other than some slight amusement at my own acquiescence in something I knew so little about. I emerged from the treatment as though having in some way passed through fire, a rite of initiation if ever there was one.

Acupuncture, and all that it has taught me about the human being in health and ill-health, has so dominated my life since that first day that I see now that such an overwhelming shift in orientation demanded some such significant event to mark its arrival. I also, I now understand, needed proof in myself of what acupuncture could do, and I could have received no more overwhelming proof than I did. For I woke the day after my first treatment as though emerging into a new world. The light seemed brighter, the colours clearer. I felt as though the grass on which I walked was connecting me through its roots to the earth beneath as though for the first time. I became aware of lines passing through me to the world around me and nature outside in a way I had never experienced before.

I had gone ostensibly for help with a physical condition. I was to find my treatment leading me into the much deeper, richer areas within me, those of my soul. To have followed this thread leading to treatment of my body and to have found it beckoning towards this deeper world is a path many of my patients still tread when they come to me, unaware, as I was then, of the awe-inspiring depth and beauty of the new world which will be opened to them. A patient of mine told me recently, 'I didn't realize when I came for treatment that I would move to such a different level of experience.'

What was it within me that thus deeply responded to my acupuncture treatment, and by such simple means effected such a profound transformation of understanding? A year later, tantalized by these mysterious questions, I started upon my study of acupuncture, and it was then that I began slowly to make my way towards a concept of the human soul which placed it so triumphantly and profoundly within a cosmic context, setting it down against the giant backcloth of the universe.

There was something infinitely satisfying in so suddenly beginning to perceive that I and the world outside me, of which I had until then been so unaware, stood in close and harmonious relation to one another. Later, when I started to study acupuncture, I was to learn that just as that world bowed to the pressures of the seasons and the years so, too, did I. It is upon the recognition of this simple and profound fact that acupuncture is based, believing as it does that a single thread is drawn through the universe along which is strung all that is, and whatever and whoever pulls upon that thread pulls upon all. I rise with the tide and fall as it ebbs. I move with the moon and dance with the sun. I blow with the wind and glisten with the rain. I freeze with the cold and melt with the heat. All that is outside me presses upon me, working within me and moulding who and what I am.

Now with my first acupuncture treatment I felt a jolt of reconnection, like the coupling of a train, as that thread winding through everything tugged gently at me, reaffirming its presence. As I walked upon the earth I seemed to have entered upon a new relationship with it, as though a veil had been removed through which I had until then perceived what was around me. There was a new clarity to my vision. The things I saw outside me and the things I saw inside me started to take on sharper focus. I became aware of the connecting ropes tying me to the world.

I found that I was standing at an intersection, with energy streaming towards me from the outermost reaches of space, channelling itself through me, like sand in an hour-glass, before pouring out again towards those far-distant places. I was to find that the cycle of that vast cosmic energy continues inside me. I am inextricably bound, by my breath alone, to the workings of the universe. I now know that, like the individual cells in my body, I cannot escape the pull of the whole.

Each life is the focal point of energies which pour through us from the cosmos, the result of a brief coalescing of these energies within our physical frame. A vast and unending play of forces swirls around us, drawing us into its infinite dance. And from its pull we cannot escape, for it melts the apparently firm edges we believe our bodies to have, making of them a place where we and the cosmos interplay. The point of intersection, where the forces of the universe bear down their great weight upon this tiny body of ours, is our skin, this delicate container, housing not only our body but our soul. This thin integument provides the merest shadow of a dividing line between the cosmos and our soul, receiving that wondrous flow of energy binding us to the great universe beyond.

Brought up as we are in the West with a model which sees this body as a fixed physical form, it is sometimes difficult, even for acupuncturists, to transform that solid image into the delicately billowing shimmer of energy, so subtly responding to the slightest pressure upon it, which we now know it to be. Nothing stands alone. All things flow and merge into one another, caught up in the ebb and flow of the great tides of the universe. The very blood in our veins responds to their call, rising and falling as the moon beckons. The air of the universe is recycled eternally through us. We breathe the air that our ancestors exhaled so many aeons ago, and what we breathe out will be there to give life to our children's children.

And the cycle of this vast cosmic energy continues within us, as the power that makes the universe wheel upon itself unto infinity plays itself out within us as our life's energy. Inside and outside, so apparently disconnected, are one, the dividing line between them no more than the faintest barrier, allowing to things their distinct and separate forms. Thus the life we lead here on earth is but the result of the fusion of these energies within this body of ours. Our body then becomes for a lifetime the flexible and delicate container within which our soul pursues its wanderings.

My first treatment had indeed become a rite of passage, an initiation all my own and without forewarning, into a new world. This was a world which introduced me to a new approach not just to health but to life. The needles, inserted into what I later discovered were called acupuncture points, had made contact with a network of intercommunications of infinite complexity. This network, I was to learn, brought me into relationship with the cadences of the natural world outside, of day and night and of the seasons and all that lay beyond me.

What was inside me, which I know as the organs of my body and its functions, was connected to what lay outside me by such tight bands that the dividing line I had thought to exist between myself and what I was not no longer existed. With little surprise, I was later to learn that the philosophical assumptions on which acupuncture is based are now reflected in those of modern physics which agrees with the ancient Chinese that a finger raised by me here on earth will affect infinitesimally the vast sweep of the most distant constellation in furthermost space.

I find this a surprisingly comforting thought, for I feel now that I belong. Tiny and insignificant though I might feel myself to be, yet I am necessary. I have a part to play, a function to perform.

So here, then, I was presented with my body, transformed into some unfamiliar object, harbouring forces which connected it to my soul, and beyond that, as I was to find, to the vast powers of the cosmos. I grew to understand that I was part of the natural forces around me, a product of a universal source of energy which creates out of itself everything that exists. I was to learn that the forces which flow to form body and soul are manifestations of the same source of energy which informs the whole universe. From the smallest flea to the blackest hole out there in deepest space, everything is a function of the balance of these forces.

Acupuncture's great contribution to human knowledge has been to recognize the physical body as the vessel within which these forces constantly interplay, and to have understood that the body sings a person's soul much as the aboriginal songlines sing the contours of Australia. Weaving their way around my body are energy lines, like ley lines, which sing me. These interconnect and intersect at all depths, drawing together the most distant parts of my body, providing a map which, if read properly, gives a true picture not only of my body but of my soul.

Some slight perception of this was given me by my response to my first treatment, an awesome first pointer to what I was later to draw together, more painstakingly, over the years to form my own understanding of the philosophical foundations and implications of my study of acupuncture. A needle inserted in a point on my body thus proved to me that it had the power to affect my vision of myself and of the world in which that self existed. Now indeed my curiosity was aroused, and turned me in the direction of investigating how what I experienced as a result of treatment could have occurred. What was this thing called acupuncture? Thus started my years of study, first only as a curious student, intent merely on finding out, before this turned, inevitably I now see, into my determination to apply these new-found insights to practice.

What I could not know at the time was that I had alighted upon the one branch of acupuncture which was so deeply able to satisfy my striving to find my soul, for it recognizes that soul above all else as the focus of its concern. And here, too, that guiding hand whose existence and benevolence I now no longer doubt led me unerringly towards what was right for me. The branch of acupuncture I had found my way towards is called five element acupuncture.

Many years on, I became the principal of a school of acupuncture which I founded, and still as curious as I was after my first treatment to explore what acupuncture does and can do, and as enthusiastic to unfold its potential to as wide an audience as possible, both through my students and, now here, to my readers.

The quest for our own identity

The reception room in my practice has a number of books for patients to read as they wait. They are mostly on subjects I think they will be interested in, such as acupuncture and general health. I also add a few books of more general interest, among them books on astrology. When I first started in practice, I expected patients to reach first for the acupuncture books, but to my surprise they do not. They eventually pick these books up, but it is the astrology books they open first, and these have been the only books that have ever disappeared.

What makes my patients so interested in astrology, and so keen, almost avid, to dip into these books? I asked several of them, and they all told me the same thing, 'I think I will learn to understand myself better.' They believe that these books contain answers to some secret knowledge about themselves and their fellow human beings which eludes them. Ultimately they are looking for answers to that great question, 'Who am I?'

This quest for self-knowledge and self-understanding appears to be something uniquely human, and one which no other living creature seems to share. It implies, too, when looked at carefully, further questions, 'What am I on this earth for? Has my life a purpose? What do we believe to be the purpose of any life? Do we, indeed, think it has a purpose at all? And, if so, how can we determine what that purpose is?'

An attempt to answer such profound questions might appear to sit uneasily within the framework of something like acupuncture, and yet I have found that I have had to seek my own answers to just such questions, if I am to practise my art as acupuncturist to the highest level. For if this impetus to acquire self-knowledge is seen, as it must be, as one of our innate impulses, it has a bearing on any therapy which aims to restore a human being to health. To my surprise, too, when I first encountered acupuncture, this quest for self-knowledge, though hidden beneath the search for relief from physical or emotional pain, became in most cases the focus of a patient's treatment.

So why do people come for acupuncture treatment? All want something to change, feel they need help in achieving this change and are looking outside themselves for this help. They may initially be unclear what it is they really want help for, but they will be coming because at some level they are not feeling well. Feeling well allows us to function without thinking of our well-being, except in those rare heightened states when we become aware of contentment flowing through us. Those things inside us which need to work to keep us healthy fulfil their allotted tasks. Lung, heart, legs, arms, emotions, thoughts, do what they must do, and do so in balance with the others. Like a well-tuned engine, all our parts whirr away as a harmonious whole. We are at one with our body and soul, and body and soul get on with things unnoticed.

Well-being is a state we take so for granted that we are affronted when it is threatened. Only then does growing unease force us to contemplate the state of our own health. When ill-health strikes in this way, this scene of harmony and order turns into a place where disharmony and disorder reign, becoming a battlefield for opposing forces. Pain and discomfort of all kinds start to appear, claiming our attention and demanding that we do something to help. Some shift in the balance of things has occurred to make the harmonious thus inharmonious, turned ease into unease and finally into disease. Why does this happen?

In Western pathology textbooks, there are very few references to any ultimate cause for many of the diseases they list, beyond those of obvious environmental or genetic origin. We know why miners get asbestosis or why smokers suffer from lung cancer, but we know next to nothing about why those other, far larger groups of illnesses make their appearance, such as multiple sclerosis or the many other forms of cancer. We know remarkably little, too, about the mechanisms which lead us to suffer even the mildest headache. All of these seem to attack one or other of us apparently spontaneously and at random. Nor, surprisingly, does this seem to bother the Western medical mind.

To the ancient Chinese, whose philosophy underpins acupuncture, such an apparent inability to create some link to an ultimate causal factor would appear incomprehensible for being in some way unordered. A view of life which acknowledges the arbitrary in this way is alien to a philosophy which sees pattern wherever it looks. If this pattern and order are disturbed, there must be a cause to this disturbance, and this is seen as originating in some infringement of the laws by which nature, in its widest sense, operates. Viewed thus, nature has cosmic overtones.

All things, including the human being, each in our tiny way, are thus manifestations of cosmic order. Illness of any kind, at any level of body or soul, appears as disorder and disharmony, and is seen as some infringement of this cosmic pattern. The aim of all treatment is to re-establish this order, set the pattern right again. How far this is possible will depend upon how entrenched any imbalance is.

This makes for a medicine of hope, offering patients the possibility of re-establishing that underlying pattern which illness has disturbed. The arbitrary appears banished. There is a reason to things which it is the acupuncturist's duty to unravel. And unravelling, as of a skein wound tight, and often knotted, is an apt metaphor for the acupuncturist's work, for the pattern to a person's life, and thus to his ill-health, lies hidden, often buried beneath the accumulations of years of imbalance. An ill patient can be seen as a garden overgrown with weeds and requiring careful husbandry to reveal outlines long obliterated and to coax life from plants long gone to seed.

And the weeds which have sprung up deep within our soul are those with the deepest roots, clinging most tenaciously and bringing with them despair and hopelessness. These, above all, we need to address if we are to help our patients back to health, and these, too, acupuncture addresses, for it makes no distinction between the sufferings of the body and those of the soul, seeing both as different manifestations of the same distress.

To the Chinese mind, the patterns underlying everything form part of a profound and carefully elaborated view of the world which sees all things as drawn together into a cohesive whole. In so doing, it knits each of us tightly into the mesh of all things, and thereby makes significant what to a Western mind is often insignificant. Illness viewed from this perspective becomes a tiny tear in the fabric of the universe, which the acupuncturist with his needle will attempt to knit together again. It is no arbitrary occurrence, but springs always from a cause which can be defined in Chinese medical terms, and thus potentially can also be put right by practices, such as acupuncture, which work within this philosophical framework.

These apparently abstract philosophical concepts therefore form the structure underlying a very practical system of medicine, reflecting in its internal cohesion that image of wholeness, which is the ultimate goal of human life. Ill-health, a movement away from harmony to disharmony, from the wholeness of health to the fragmentation of illness, is a sign of some weakening in the forces of wholeness. Viewed from the standpoint of this philosophy, an acupuncturist's task is thus to make the broken whole again, to restore harmony to the disharmonious.

This understanding of the nature of ill-health, apparently so simple, allows for the construction of a highly complex tracking system enabling the most subtle interferences with the natural, healthy flow of energies through us to be detected at any stage, and, once detected, to be adjusted using a sophisticated armoury of subtle therapeutic interventions. A turn of the needle, in the right place, at the right time and for the right reason, can ease an arthritic joint, reduce blood pressure, still a troubled mind, or do all these together. Once such adjustments have been made, the same procedures can be used to resist further pressures towards imbalance, turning acupuncture into a highly effective form of preventive medicine.

The cadence of the universe

The pattern of things which the Chinese recognized is expressed in terms of profound symbols. The cosmos, and all within it, existing forever beyond time and space, is known as the Dao, that which encompasses everything. The Dao is the universe unmanifest, the universe before the Big Bang. As imperfect, finite mortals who are born to die, we can only imperfectly comprehend or describe the Dao, for it is all that is perfect, eternal and infinite. Being beyond our comprehension, the most transcendental of words are needed to describe it, and I make no claim to be able to do what only the greatest poets and musicians can achieve. Perhaps it is enough to describe it as the All, out of which emerges time and space and eventually matter, and with matter each tiny human being.

Beneath and beyond the cyclical processes of change and transformation in which we engage, body and soul, as the necessary condition of all life, beneath and beyond the impermanent and transitory, all things are seen to emerge from a state of cosmic unity, the Dao, and to return to it once their temporary forms have exhausted their span, individual manifestations of matter and life being seen always only as fragments of the whole.

At its moment of manifestation, the Dao breaks apart into two opposing forces. To this conflict of opposites, this cosmic balancing-act, the Chinese have given the name of the dance of yin and yang, that dance of opposites forever held apart and forever striving to embrace one another. This creates the great duality of all things, their positive and their negative poles, the two arms of a balance, eternally seeking to merge again as one into the Dao. Thus the two poles of an electrical current, the inside and outside of everything, the light and the dark, the male and the female, back and front, good and evil, the thing that is and the thing that it is not. To exist, all things live in a state of oscillating duality in which yin strives with yang as night strives with day and positive with negative, a battle neither side can win, else all manifest things will disintegrate into the unmanifest, disappearing into endless night. And out of the resulting tension there develops a dynamic thrust, robbing us of rest and denying us the comforts of inertia.

My hand here writing this shows me its yang side, its back. My palm, hidden, as all yin things would like to be, encloses my pen. I have to turn my hand and open it before I can see the surface of the palm. As soon as I relax my attention, my hand curls slightly inwards again, enclosing my palm again, which is once more hidden from my sight. The yin aspect of my hand seeks, however instinctively, the dark and the hidden. Its yang aspect is happy to reveal itself, and yet both yin and yang, palm and back of hand, need each other to exist.

This is a simple but profound illustration of yin and yang. I could just as easily have chosen any one of an infinite number of illustrations, since everything that is manifest is only manifest through the union of yin with yang. In that sense, all in the universe is twofold, dual, itself and its reverse. Implicit in one thing is thus its opposite.

Yin and yang, passing their energy to and fro, as some juggler a ball from hand to hand, need a further impetus for the movement necessary for time and space to occur. In turn, they convert their power into the forces which make change and development possible. These are five phases in the eternal cycling of all things from start to finish, drawn out each from the womb of yin and yang, and each adding to that oscillating movement the potential to move forward and thus to change. As the Dao breaks apart to form matter, so yin and yang divide into forces which give to all things those movements which make life possible. They create the impetus for each seed to form, bud, blossom, wither and ultimately die. In our bodies, they create differing organs each with their different functions in this cycle of birth, renewal and death. We call these five phases the five elements.

Each of these forces brings its own specific creative quality to the forward impetus they together impart to yin and yang, and each in turn, like spokes of a wheel, connects to the next in some eternal cycle of movement, drawing life from the lifeless and, in that cycle's final rotation, bringing death. Yin and yang, the opposing forces, and the five elements, the forces moving us forward, fuse to form all living things, and ultimately each tiny fragment of human life we each represent.

All things in the universe dance to the beat of these five forces, which hold within their infinite grasp the span of all that lives and dies and is born again. Of the moving force guiding this hand we can have but the dimmest concept, so clouded are our perceptions, but this is the force which directs the flow of those great constellations wheeling in infinite space and the brief flutter of a bird's wings. In an attempt to find symbols sufficiently simple and profound to bear the weight of all that is, the Chinese conceived of this force in terms of the natural world they saw around them, for what greater forces can we think of than those to which we owe life? And thus they described this cycle of birth to death as passing through five phases to which they gave the simple, everyday names of Wood, Fire, Earth, Metal and Water. Each of these forces has its own clearly defined task, but all are interdependent and interlocking, together forming the dense canvas of the universe.

These five symbols can condense themselves down to the tiny dimensions of the energies flowing through each of us, widen out as though in the growing arc of a spotlight to include the planet's seasonal cadences, or extend far beyond us to encompass the forces which dictate the flow of the great universe beyond. At each of these levels, from the human to the cosmic, they trace a progression from birth to death to rebirth, plotting an endless and continuous circle of life and containing with their infinite grasp the alpha and omega of all that exists.

The totality of the energy by which we live and by which we die is held within this five-fold grasp. Thus there is a part of us which owes allegiance to the energies of what we call the element Wood, another to those of Fire, another to those of Earth, another to those of Metal and another to those of Water. Together these flow within us to form the complete cycle of our life.

The five great energies, those fingers of the giant hand holding all in its grasp, create life in its totality as they create all things under the sun and beyond the sun. They form the very cells of each organ and define the organs' functions. What in acupuncture are known as the deep and superficial pathways of energy, the meridians, dissect the body at all levels, and can only be understood properly if we allow these lines to spread and splay out until they form an intricate network of energy creating with their actions the physical structures and the functions of those structures which we call by the names of the organs. Our energy is drawn from the surface to the deep and returned from there to the surface, at its depth creating the organs themselves, and at its surface replenishing its energy from the endless supply pouring to it from the cosmos. Only at death does this awesome inhalation and exhalation process, mirrored by similar processes in all the organs, falter and eventually break down, with death occurring at the moment of disconnection, when something, some exhaustion of the energetic flow necessary to maintain life, breaks the rhythmic cadences which generate life.

Enmeshing to form the tight strands of energy which turn our cells into ligaments or bones, connective tissue or blood vessel, the elements transform the first tiny cell of us into the ever more complex manifestations of advanced life to which each human being bears witness. And just as we are simply replications of the one original cell of the embryo into the innumerable cells of our maturity, so the elements, fusing their efforts to produce that first cell, continue their work within the increasingly intricate framework of the mature body. They represent the cosmos manifesting within each human being, the power of five on an infinite scale replicated within every one of us.

These five phases represent the movement inherent in all things, the processes by which change and development are made possible. They cause life to unfold from the single cell of its beginnings towards its point of maturity and decline. They create time, making all that is into what it will become, and then converting it into what has been. And specifically, in the human being, which is what interests us here, they manifest themselves as the different processes involved in the formation, maintenance and development of all aspects of our being. The elements are the body's agents of transformation, representing each a different phase in the cycle of life. And it is these forces which acupuncture taps.

Together they are life in its totality. Their different functions at all these levels combine to form a complex, ultimately unfathomable tissue of interactions from which emerges a form, a shape, the unique being which is each one of us. From the bones which shape us, to the flesh upon these bones, to the arteries feeding the flesh and bones, all are a function of the elements' work. They are those processes by which our bodies come to life, grow and eventually decay, each element bringing into being different organs and energy pathways, and having each its own physical sphere of influence.

And at a deeper, less physical level within us, they exercise control over those aspects within us which endow us with our soul, determining as much what makes us think the way we do as what makes us laugh and cry. All that vast range of our life which we call by the name of thoughts, emotions, desires, our deep craving for what lies beyond and above us, all this, too, owes its existence and its health to the power of the elements within us. Emotionally, therefore, the elements point us towards what are regarded as the five great emotions, anger, joy, sympathy, grief or fear, each with its own needs, that of a desire for structure, for love, for nourishment, for respect or for reassurance.

The ancient Chinese developed a very sophisticated understanding of the functioning of the human being, body and soul, along the scale from a state of good health to one of ill-health, and formulated a cohesive, internally consistent system of medicine whose principal tools of diagnosis and treatment are the fundamental philosophical concepts of yin/yang and the five elements. When we grow ill, yin and yang no longer balance each other and the five elements lose their ability to circle harmoniously within us. These forces of cohesion then turn into forces of disintegration, for the dividing-line between a world capable of sustaining life or a barren planet, between the earth warmed by the welcome heat of summer or scorched by blistering heat-waves, is very finely drawn. The whole universe walks upon a tightrope balancing in its two hands the weight of opposing forces. We live our lives pulled between positive and negative poles.

The processes of growth which add ring upon perfect ring to the trunk of a tree can be seen as symbols of the action of the elements in the cycle of nature outside. Layer upon layer of new life is added as the tree grows over the years, and yet no break in the rings can be detected. The transition from one phase of growth to the next takes place smoothly, each slipping imperceptibly into the next, as the tree thickens and ages. We too grow and age and die in rhythm with the flow of the elements through us.

And there are many rhythms to which we are subjected. There is the rhythm that leads from our birth to our death, and the rhythm of the days, the seasons and the years. And then there are the rhythms within us, of the drawing of breath, of the throbbing of the heart, of the movement of the blood. The actions by which the body recycles over the years the very substance of which it is made, sloughing off as dead skin what has served its purpose and then creating itself anew, are products of the cyclical work of the elements.

They create a rhythm to all life, as though the great lungs of the universe are breathing in and out in endless motion. And this gives us the great rhythmic contrasts, the beat of the night against the beat of the day, the beat of summer against that of winter, the beat of yin against the beat of yang, which punctuate our lives at all points.

We, too, are made of such rhythms, our bodies tiny microcosms of the great cosmic rhythm outside. The cycle of our life has its cadence, its rises and falls, its peaks and its troughs, a constant dynamic of expansion and contraction. And in this it echoes the pulse of all things, the attraction and repulsion of atom to atom, the ebb and flow of the tides, the billowing of the clouds and the great wheeling of constellations upon one another throughout deepest space. All things throb to some hidden rhythm, and all, as far as we can ever know, are born to die and be reborn in other and different groupings of the matter from which they are formed. The energy which shapes us is eternal, an unborn, undying force which coaxes out of its infinite womb the myriad forms of life which know both birth and death.

This places us under the yoke of time, and casts the shadow of its passing upon us. Time moulds all it touches into the shapes of death and renewal. It breaks up the unchanging monotony of the eternal into the individual fragments we know as cycles of hours, day, lifetimes, millennia, and gives to each its own cadence. It pulls the year to its height in summer, and flattens it beneath its winter mantle of cold. It turns us from babes in arms to the senile in our wheelchairs, ruthlessly replacing the smooth face of youth with the wrinkles of old age. It knows no mercy, for nothing can escape its tyranny.

The qualities of energy we call the elements represent differing dynamics along this cycle of life, as the seasons represent the movements which turn the years upon themselves in their endless wheeling. A different kind of energy produces the dynamic thrust which calls forth the birth of all things from that which guides these same things towards their maturity and on to their descent towards extinction. And thus the energy of all beginnings has a quality all its own which differentiates it from that of all endings, and again from all those intermediary stages which punctuate the passage from start to finish. Our morning energy differs from that of our evening, just as the deep silence of midnight finds us different from when noon's noisy bustle hustles us along. We are part of the days' turning, the seasons' change, the years' passing.

These cyclical changes are the marks branded by time upon all things. And just as the world is subject to a process of constant transformation, so each small parcel of life contained within it bears upon it its own imprint of time's passing. The rise and fall in the cadence of life is as detectable within us as without. All things obey the call of this ebb and flow, as the energy of which we are made yields, minute by minute, year by year, to the rhythms of life and death. And this beat is that of the elements, for they are life in all the stages of its becoming.

In this dynamic process, in which shifts in energy throughout the structure of the body bring about its daily, monthly, yearly ageing, different aspects of this energy predominate at different times. The rise and fall within them provides the impetus towards change to which all things are subject. In nature outside, spring energy must yield to summer energy, as summer must to autumn and autumn to winter, as the cycle of the seasons spirals onwards through the years. And so it is with our body. Its energies have their own peaks and troughs throughout the cycles of time, each type of energy assuming temporary control for a certain period of time, before handing over to the next, just as one season passes on responsibility to its successor. There is an ordered progression to the rise and fall in each of these energies, as each fulfils its purpose within the cycle of wholeness.

As I sit here, pen in hand, paper before me, my soul engaged, my mind attempting to find expression for that which my soul feels, my body shifting on the chair, all these different facets of my being and my doing are defined by the different qualities of the elements working their creative magic upon me. The sum of their qualities forms all that is complete in itself, a totality, whether it be the body as a whole, or any of its manifestations, the formulation of a thought, the articulation of a movement, the digestion of a meal, the growing of a hair, the shutting of an eye, the opening of a door, the expression of grief or the moral outrage we feel.

And what more appropriate, in this product of the written word, than to examine the elements as they help me formulate the very words I am trying to find to describe them? First, the start of the thought out of which will grow the word on the page, the impetus without which nothing can take root and grow, its moment of budding. Then the development, the growth to maturity, the bud bursting into full blossom, the thought now ripe with promise, its fruit, the words, ready to fall from pen to paper, and then the critical appraisal, a word added, a sentence changed, perhaps all that has been written deleted in one savage cut in the name of purity and truth, and then the moment of pause, before the process of putting thought to paper restarts with the next word. From Wood, bud, to Fire, blossom, to Earth, fruit, to Metal, evaluation, to Water, pause, the elements together lead me, step by step, to this full stop.

The guardian of the soul

We now need to turn to an acupuncture chart, familiar to many of us. Here we see lines running up and down the body indicating what we call pathways of energy, known as meridians or channels. You will see that points are marked at intervals along these lines, and these are the places at which acupuncture needles are inserted. What creates these meridians is something we can call by many names. I have chosen to call this force energy, for simplicity's sake. Its equivalent Chinese terms are qi, chi or ki. It is our life force. It is that which infuses every cell in my body with life, and when withdrawn renders these same cells lifeless.

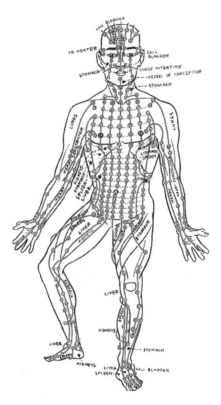

What we notice immediately in this chart is a powerful sense of symmetry and balance. The shaping the meridians impart to the body draw its lines together into a harmonious whole, from toe to fingertip. What cannot be shown in this two-dimensional representation is that this ordered structure continues beneath the surface of the body, tying all parts of it together and forming an ever more complex network of interconnecting pathways, ultimately enmeshing each cell with every other cell.

A profound echo of this symmetrical image of the body is to be found in Leonardo da Vinci's pictorial representation of the body, his famous cartoon. Here we see it housed within a perfect globe, enclosed by something greater than itself which enfolds it, as though in its own embryonic sac. The body has become a wheel, with its spokes our arms and legs and its axis our trunk. In its perfect symmetry and balance, it seems poised to rotate upon itself at the slightest touch. To the ancient Chinese, this would be a pictorial representation of their own concept of the human being embedded within the cosmic order, at harmony within this cosmic order and responsive to any movement around and within it.

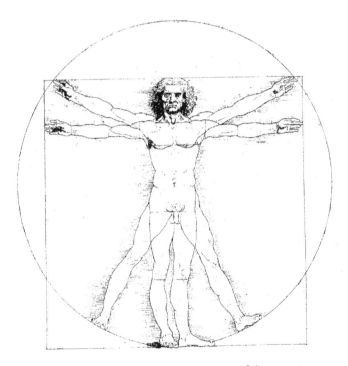

This wheeling is a symbolic representation of the cosmic energy of the Dao, yin/yang and the five elements. The Dao is the circle, without beginning or end, wheeling unto infinity, a symbol of the world in eternal unity and peace before the universe broke apart. Yin/yang is the duality which brings movement to the Dao by introducing the tension of opposites, represented by the vertical and horizontal divisions in Leonardo's cartoon. And finally, the five elements are manifestations of the forward movement introduced into all things, revealing the cadence from yin to yang, from dark to light, from night to day, from summer to winter, without which time and space, and with them life, would be impossible. These are the four limbs and the trunk in Leonardo's drawing, here motionless, but seeking only the slightest breath, absent from this cartoon, to set the perfect globe pulsing into life.

Now we need to flesh the skeleton out a little more, and we will do this by looking more closely at Leonardo's cartoon and its companion acupuncture chart. The ancient Chinese would have agreed with Leonardo that the body is symmetrically aligned. A quick glance at an acupuncture chart and a knowledge of the interconnecting pathways beneath the skin's surface will show how every part of our body, apparently so clearly defined, is linked to other far-distant parts, so that one and the same meridian feeds, for example, the eye, the mouth, the chest, the stomach, the lower abdomen, the thigh, the knee, the ankle and the toe, connecting there with another running in the opposite direction which feeds another part of the foot, the ankle and so on, until every inch of the body is enveloped in this dense network of energy lines.

And these same meridians have a role to play in the work of the lymphatic system, menstruation, mastication and much more, and also affect the inner processes of thought and emotion. All these, and a myriad of other functions, are some of the tasks of the energy flowing to and from the nose and eye, so that nose and eye then become not only the places where we breathe and see, but a repository of many other aspects of our life, any one of which can show its distress by throwing out of balance the energy along the meridians running to this area.

Viewed in this way, hay fever, sinusitis, asthma or the common cold, as well as all these deeper imbalances which burden us all, can be seen as caused by impediments to the smooth flow of energy through a part of the meridian network, which passes through the nose, mouth and head. To remove these blockages, it may not be necessary to place needles somewhere around the area of pain, for the original blockage to the energy may have occurred elsewhere along the meridian pathway, on the foot, for example, or deep within us, causing a distant part of the network to seize up. We may therefore needle the foot to clear the blocked nose or the deeper pain.

The Western scientific outlook, though increasingly aware that all energy is one, has so far failed to formulate a revised medical framework which takes account of this newly gained knowledge. Here Western medicine lags behind Western physics for some reason, probably because an acceptance of the oneness of all things will threaten what the Chinese mind would consider to be the arbitrary divisions of Western physiology, and the even more arbitrary accentuation of the importance of the body at the cost of attention to the soul within that body.

This is not to devalue the amazing advances Western medicine has made, and continues to make, in treating many of the ills of that body, particularly where drastic interventions are called for. And yet doctors' surgeries are full of patients crying out for help for that vast range of non-specific illnesses the doctors themselves know not how to treat. To one trained in an approach to health which recognizes the unity of the human being, those odd feelings of malaise, unease, unhappiness, intermittent aches and pains, do not represent the puzzle they are for Western medicine, but are an accurate statement of some imbalance somewhere within the body or soul of the patient. And such an imbalance can be traced to its source as distress within one or more of the elements, and treated by adjusting the energy flowing within this element or elements. This adjustment is done by means of an acupuncture needle.

How does this body, itself so limited in form and size, cope with harbouring such vast and intangible powers as are those of our soul? The constant expansion of these powers, created by the intense internal developments the human being is capable of, exerts its own pressure upon our physical envelope. Like some balloon whose surface reflects the tension of air within it, the contours of the body, in much more complex fashion, reflect the state of the soul enfolded within its grasp, making it a living symbol of those inner powers. Fused together for a lifetime into the shape which is each one of us, this makes of the physical body always more than its mere material presence.

It is, then, not some fixed outline, irrevocably stamped with the template of an individual life, its shape and being as firmly determined as any stone. It is susceptible to the force of pressures working upon it from within which have so deep an influence upon the physical framework within which they shelter that they have the power to stamp upon our faces their lines of worry, upon our ankles their swellings and upon our backs the burden of our distresses.

What defines the contours of my body? What places upon my face my expression and imposes upon the frame of my bones the shape which makes of me something energetic or tired or sad? What gives the way I hold myself or move my hands its imprint of anger or fear or hesitation? The body is a living, dynamic mould, absorbing into itself the shapes of the emotions, the imprint of the feelings, and turns the softness of its loving where necessary into harsh defence against attack. It is a fluid symbol of our being, and yet we see it as solid. By some subtle osmosis, this thing, though tightly sheathed in its grip of muscle and flesh, can reflect an infinite variety of emotions upon its apparently harsh and unyielding frame.

And where better to start this exploration of acupuncture than with what is apparently the site of its first action, this body into which the acupuncture needle is inserted. Perhaps, too, living as I do in a Western world and writing for what I assume is predominantly a Western audience, it would be as well to start with the body, as Western medicine does. The physician prescribes drugs for it to take, whilst the surgeon uses his instruments to cut into it. The acupuncturist, too, inserts fine needles into its surface and applies healing herbs to it. To this extent, both systems of medicine direct their treatment at the same place. Where they diverge, however, and so very strongly, too, as almost to be at different ends of a spectrum, is in their concept of what that body represents.

Years back, before I learnt about acupuncture, my body seemed so simple an object. It was something I could touch and see, a thing out there, scarcely different from any rock or stone strewn around me on the ground. It appeared to have an existence apart from me, a life of its own which I could observe with those other parts of me, my mind and my soul. Sometimes it would sicken unexpectedly, and then it would force its way into the foreground of my thoughts because of its unease. At other times it functioned so smoothly that I took it for granted, accepting its favours ungratefully and as though by right. Nowhere in this picture did I link to this physical envelope of mine those deeper aspects of my being which encompassed my emotional and spiritual life.

And when disease struck, I looked to others to repair me, as though my body was a vehicle needing service at the garage. Illness was something that attacked my body, an alien presence to be repulsed and vanquished, an invader from outside, a thing, yet another to add to all those other things of matter which formed what I thought of as the world. And like some machine, my body appeared to be dependent not upon the environment in which I lived, but upon the skills of the mechanic and the availability of spare parts. The miracles of modern medicine, the joint replacements, transplant surgery, replacement drugs, all appeared to me to be confirmation of a belief that nature had failed and that the man-made was the only thing that could now help.

It is difficult for me to remember myself now as I was then, but looking back it seems at some level that I regarded mankind as knowing more than nature, for did not the only medicine I then knew about assure me that it had to step in at every opportunity to repair what nature had apparently broken? From there, it was only a dangerously short step to the belief that we always know better than nature, with its implication that to leave things to natural forces is somehow to return to the primitive.

I was a child of my time, a time of science, which revelled in all that it could do, with no hint yet of the problems of pollution or whisper of drug side-effects. The discoveries of medicine would cure all, we thought. And I was steeped in this tradition, my father a doctor, the wards of a hospital a familiar place. The secret of health was out there in the hands of others. All disease must yield before this array of expertise, as we headed towards a future resplendent with health.

And this was an approach which I continued to take for granted until my first encounter with acupuncture. It was only then that I started to question many of the assumptions about health with which I grew up.

What I gradually discovered was that, whereas the Western view of the body is limited almost entirely to what is accessible to physical analysis, acupuncture regards the body, not as an end in itself, but as a channel or container. The body becomes an entrance to the deeper, inner world of the soul. And the soul is not regarded, as in the West, as being somehow vaguely independent of the body, an elusive quality floating haphazardly within its confines, as though almost untouched by, and leaving untouched, the complex functions of the body, but as an integral part of its workings, interconnected at every level with the physical structure within which it is embedded.

For body cannot move without its companion soul, just as soul needs a physical dwelling-place in which to manifest itself.

The body as portrait of the soul

To accept such a widening of our concept of the body requires a leap of imagination and understanding that many of us in the West find threatening, brought up as we are to isolate our bodies from all but the physical, and to banish the rest of us to remote regions, such as religion or psychiatry. Some slight acknowledgement of the concept of the whole person is occasionally made, and then we talk of psychosomatic or stress-induced illness, but with no clear idea of what this really means and almost in derogatory terms, as though such conditions are thereby somehow less than worthy of our full attention. What is lacking is any vision of that thread which ties the apparently disconnected parts of us together to form the whole we so patently are.

Acupuncture accepts as self-evident the chain of cause and effect which passes from body to soul and from soul to body. It sees the body as the envelope within which our inner being finds its physical expression, and understands that illness of the body can arise as much, if not more, from inner distress as from purely physical causes. And, beyond this, it sees each of us as being an integral part of forces outside ourselves, a tiny thread in the vast web of cosmic life, our health and ill-health a function of the balance of these forces both within and without.

Viewed from acupuncture's perspective, our body can be seen to flow, its edges softened by the passage of those streams of energy which form our cells, changing shape, succumbing to the pressure of pain, hardening to bitterness and anger, yielding to the warm delights of love. It is the physical symbol of the soul. It is infinitely flexible, swift to adapt to prevent annihilation, marvellously complex in its mechanisms, beautifully balanced in its proportions, the living work of a creator's art, most wondrous guardian of our soul. It makes available to us an opening, a way in to the deep landscape of our inner world, becoming a medium through which our inner powers of thought and emotion are accessible to intervention. It is then the visible, palpable place where the invisible, impalpable levels of mind and spirit can find their physical expression.

At each moment it is a living, changing portrait of the soul, and visible upon it, in every outline, is the state of the soul's being, for the soul will paint upon it happiness and pain, laughter and desolation. It will mould its contours, sculpting into the flesh and the bones with the chisel of our fate the forms which our life imposes upon us. We are stamped with the soul's template, the body forever bearing the imprint of our emotions and thoughts, just as it offers a physical response to the demands made upon it.

This secret and hidden part of us is both tender and tough. An elusive guest, slipping unseen on its wanderings within us, yet it dominates all that we do, hidden master of the ramparts and fortifications of the body which shelters it. So strong is its presence, so remorseless the pressure it exerts upon this body, that our very bones, so apparently hard and inflexible, are forced to yield, bowing and crooking themselves in response to its demands. For when our soul succumbs to pressure, our body, too, must reflect this defeat. Our backs will bend, our vertebrae grind, our shoulders hunch, as life tightens its grip upon us.

To ask of the body that it represent only itself, and not those other deeper parts of us, our mind and spirit, is to reduce it to no more than the shadow of its true significance, and to ignore its true function. A body at peace and at ease with itself reflects a soul thus at peace and at ease. A body contorted with pain reflects a soul thus contorted with pain. A back will stoop if work has buckled it, and this stoop becomes a physical imprint upon our body's shape. But what if the burdens of our emotional life weigh down upon it? Then, too, it may bend, bowing low before pressures greater than the mere physical. If a face can show in its lines of anxiety and frowns of anger how we are feeling, then the whole body, too, must similarly offer itself as an emotional register. Perhaps the face, that most plastic and malleable part of us, will reveal its emotional imprint most markedly, but echoes will be found even in those least flexible parts of us, our bony places. Just as our faces will etch with the pains of life, so will our fingers clench and our toes tighten with the strain of anger and distress.

Our outermost layer, our skin, can be seen as a multi-faceted doorway, its major entrances those apertures we use for breathing, nourishment, excretion and reproduction, with a myriad of less visible key-holes, our pores, through which energy is inhaled and exhaled. And these apertures open inside us upon a complex landscape of tissue and bone, a densely structured edifice whose varied parts have developed each their own highly differentiated function whilst maintaining an astonishing unity of purpose. All parts, lung, knee, brain, liver, flesh, all work, except in illness, with the same object in mind, the maintenance of the whole.

Buried deep within ourselves in mysterious and inaccessible places, into which the eye cannot penetrate, lie the organs of the body. Over liver and heart, kidney and spleen arches the protective awning of our skin, hiding all but our surface from view. Only those few openings necessary for life pierce this closed container. Despite its apparent fragility, the wondrous protection of man's outer casing is sufficiently resistant to withstand a lifetime's knocks and blows.

It holds us in its protective embrace, flexibly moulding itself around the intricate pathways of nerve and blood, flowing over the firm contours of muscle and bone, opening itself to welcome inside it, through pore and mouth and nose, the gifts of life the cosmos showers upon us, and closing down to defend us from attack. It is like some sensitive antenna turning towards the pulses of cosmic life which throb around it. Our skin gives us our boundaries, turning its outer face outwards to confront the unknown stretching out into infinity beyond its reach, and its inner face inwards to watch over those hidden parts of us, which human eye was never intended to see, so precious and private are their functions.

The wonder is that as acupuncturists we have been given the means to penetrate beneath this surface, and intrude upon the delicate balance of these intricately interwoven energies within us. The needle, superficially breaching the body's ramparts, sends signals to every cell stimulating all to action where action is needed, repelling invaders which bear disease from without, and on the lookout for disturbance from within. Our energy channels, the meridians, mapped for us in infinite detail since the beginning of recorded time, bear their life-giving energy from the depths to our surface, here for the first time becoming accessible to touch and to the needle. It is here where the cosmos presses against the soft barrier of our body that the energies which reflect that constant and creative tension between the world inside us and the world outside us offer themselves to us for modification.

This cosmic flow through and out of us again is defined in very precise terms. An intricate network of energy pathways has been traced throughout our body, highways along which this energy streams out to the furthermost regions of the body. Each meridian has its own specific function within the body's overall energy pattern, and together they form a dense, interlocking web of energy penetrating from the surface of our body deep within us, and feeding every cell in the body. This network is a reception point for the energy flowing towards us, as we take in and process cosmic energy in the form of air and food, and return it again to the cosmos as waste products.

The network interlinks at many places with pathways running deeper within the body, forming a fine mesh interweaving every cell in every part of the body with every other cell elsewhere. The superficial network can be seen highlighted by certain forms of photography, is visible to a highly practised eye and palpable to a highly practised hand. And the meridians feed with energy not only the deeper levels of our body but also of our soul.

To the acupuncturist, the body's demarcation-line of skin is the site of all his work. No need for us to delve deeper within the body than its surface, for towards that surface pour, from outside, all the energies of the universe and, from inside, all the energies feeding our every cell. Their meeting-place is thus not the too, too solid flesh we might choose to think it, but a delicate and porous membrane breathing in cosmic life.

The whole energy network can be likened to a central heating system, with the organs its radiators, the meridians its pipes, and the heart its pump, supplying not only our physical needs but also our souls with what they need to survive. This energy does not merely pass through each cell, as the meridians seen on acupuncture charts appear to run through our bodies, but is the energy which forms each cell. Unlike a central heating system which passes through the house warming it with its network of pipes, the meridian system not only feeds the body, but forms it. The energy of the liver does not merely pass through the liver, like some visitor to a site, but constitutes the liver. We are the energies of the elements.

The organs, in Chinese medicine, are therefore regarded, not only as those physical structure we know so much about, but as having specific mental and spiritual characteristics of their own. The heart is that which pulsates and pumps blood around the body, but it is also regarded as more than this; it is the place where resides our capacity to love and to live in joy. The liver in Chinese medicine is that which filters blood and detoxifies poisons, but it is also the place where resides our capacity to structure our life, and the seat of the emotion we call anger.

Our organs are the elements' sites of greatest concentration. As the tiny embryo pushes its boundaries outwards in the womb, growing limbs, fingers, toes and all the features with which it emerges into life, the elements extend their work along networks of ever-increasing complexity. Different energies bring into being each different part of us, a heart energy producing the heart, a stomach energy the stomach, a bladder energy the bladder, and a liver energy the liver. These differentiated forms of energy do not only remain localized within the organ which gives them their name, but traverse the body throughout the meridian network. The heart dispatches its own energy through this network to do its work around the body with the aid of the heart meridians, as we know it does through the system of blood vessels, just as that of the spleen moves along other pathways, the spleen meridians, to perform the specific functions which are designated those of the spleen.

The body thus represents a miraculous explosion of energy outwards from the single cell at the moment of our creation to the intricate structures of a fully developed human being. As these cells cluster and multiply, they place themselves under a complex system of organization in which each individual part upholds the integrity of the whole by fulfilling a particular function geared to ensure its proper development. It is thus that the individual organs develop their own functions, and all parts of us, such as muscles and nerves, assume specific responsibilities. Without such a meticulous division of labour within us, we would be unable to develop the complex features characterizing the mature human being of today which give us our capacity for advanced thought and deep feeling.

Within our first cell is the genetic material which determines our final shape, as does the plan within a bud determine the shape of the tree it is to become. The energy forming the cell, its genetic energy, provides the cell with the impetus to divide and cluster in specific ways to allow a heart to develop, a hand to emerge, a brain to unfold. And locked into this heart, this hand, this brain, are those energy pulses which formed them. Interlinked in a tight web, these circulate in a beautifully concerted dance of energy throughout our body to maintain life.

The acupuncture chart and Leonardo's cartoon show the human being as a body. What they cannot depict is what that body contains which animates it, gives it its soul. Woven into the actions of the elements within the body are those which feed our soul, and they, too, are influenced at these sites along the body, and, in turn, will influence the health or ill-health of the body. The aspects of our physical body which we differentiate into organs and functions are thus given in Chinese medicine mysterious companions, those differentiated expressions of our soul, our emotions and spiritual aspirations, without which, according to this philosophy, no discussion of these physical structures can take place. The emotions are to be seen not simply as attributes attached to the elements, like barnacles to a rock, but as an organic expression of their deepest nature. We recognize this implicitly, but often without appreciating the significance of what we are saying, when we cry out that we are broken-hearted, for surely we do not think that our physical heart is breaking apart? It is our heart's soul which is calling out in pain.

In Western medicine, we have no means of linking this pain with our physical heart. In Chinese medicine, the pathway of energy which affects our physical heart, the heart meridian, running from under our armpit down the inside of our arm to the tip of our little finger, in its deep wanderings below the surface of our skin touches upon the physical organ, the heart, which we recognize from our anatomy textbooks, as well as upon its mental and spiritual companions, which no X-ray can detect, but whose presence we all tacitly assume when we talk with joy or pain of affairs of the heart. The meridian system of energy pathways locks soul into a tight embrace with the body through which it passes. Thus the angry mood with which we wait in a traffic jam will send messages of distress to the liver meridian, and therefore to the big toe, the ankle and the shinbone. This will cause our bile to rise, our eyes to glare, our hands to strum on the steering wheel, our feet to press tighter on the pedals, whilst our teeth clench at irritation at being late for an interview.

All these differing signs of distress, some of the body, some of the soul within that body, can be influenced by different means. We can learn meditation techniques to calm our frustration, humming our mantras as we sit in traffic. We can listen to soothing music to calm our nerves (and here these are both our physical nerves causing our jaw to clench, and our emotional nerves making us distressed). If we become aware that our responses to the frustrations imposed upon us by the outside world are becoming exaggerated, we can also turn outside ourselves for help, and call our acupuncturist to prevent us bursting out in road rage, or shouting at our partners.

Nature's pull towards health

My understanding of the powers of this new world of healing into which I had wandered was gradual, a slow awakening upon what was to me, at first, an alien landscape. I started out from the familiar world of physical medicine in which I had grown up, the world of my body which was so reassuringly there before me, offering solid proof of my existence. I was to find this same body transformed into a shimmering mass of energy, sheltering what I now see as that deepest, most awesome part of me, my soul, and responding to the slightest pressure upon it of that soul. Ills of the body gradually melded with ills of the spirit, the familiar distinction between them now blurred. The needle, I found, could touch my soul as it so obviously touched my body, stirring that soul back to health, as it could the body.

Exactly what part the soul plays in our body's functioning is of great concern to acupuncture, in contrast to Western medicine, where the nature of this relationship, and its relevance to the health or ill-health of the body, is largely ignored, probably because it raises such disquieting questions. In the West, when the spirit is considered to be out of balance, it is said, almost dismissively, to produce that wide and vague category of illnesses labelled as stress-induced, psychosomatic, or, more succinctly, simply as mental. But, on the whole, that is as far as it goes. The close relationship acupuncture accepts sits uneasily within the tight physical framework within which Western medicine operates.

Such an approach has come to mean more to me than one which, by limiting the body rigidly to its physical role, concentrates almost entirely upon what can be physically measured and thus disregards anything which lies beyond the scope of its parameters. We can indeed choose to concentrate our attention upon the outside of things, for this is the face which is turned towards us, and thus it is possible to pause at the threshold of the physical, refusing to pass beyond that gate of skin and bone where beckon the deeper and more hidden parts of us. We can remain convinced that the physical contains the key to life's secrets. And then the body becomes a trap, deceiving us by its very solidity and apparent reality into thinking that it holds the answers to all the questions of human health, and that it is only the inadequacy of our measuring methods which have so far failed us.

But only the physical can be grasped by physical means. Science must always fall silent before that which is not physical within us, for instruments, measurers only of the measurable, cannot by their very nature grasp the immeasurable. And the realm of our soul, unlike that of our body, is immeasurable, although its effects are not. We can measure the heart beat, but can we measure what makes this same heart love? We can measure our physical being, those parts of us which appear, in life, upon the scan, and lie dissected after death upon the laboratory bench, but we cannot measure that something which transforms them into more than just the sum of their physical parts. And this quality is the spirit of life which makes us, in its presence, a person alive and functioning, and, in its absence, a corpse.

This understanding gives to the practice of acupuncture a dimension which extends far beyond the sphere of physical medicine, moving into those areas which the fields of psychotherapy and spiritual counselling call their own. Where acupuncture relates to Western medicine in its concept of the physical energies of the various organs, it relates to modern psychotherapeutic practice in its understanding of the differing emotional characteristics which together make up the human being. Where it differs from both is in the fact that, having a clear concept of the soul within the body, and accessible through the body, it can use the same treatment to treat both. Indeed, it cannot treat one level without treating the others.

In acupuncture, physical health can never be regarded as distinct from mental or spiritual health. A division between what can be analyzed by scientific methods and what, like distresses of the spirit or mental unease, cannot, is alien to it. The deep connections which it recognizes between our physical outer being and our inner being weave themselves tightly into every part of its diagnosis and treatment. It is the intimate relationship between these levels of our being whose delicate balance acupuncture accepts as being a determining factor in our health.

In diagnosing, an acupuncturist therefore makes no distinction between those ailments which appear physical in origin (a bad back, a headache) and those which appear to originate at a deeper level within us (heartache, depression, sadness, confusion), for all levels interconnect to form the one being, and all equally reveal the elements' state of balance or imbalance. Indeed, the deeper ills, by reason of their depth and importance to us, are of particular concern to us, and demand the greater focus for a practitioner.

This is often an area of acupuncture unfamiliar to many who come for treatment, for acupuncture, being apparently a physical form of treatment, using a physical needle to penetrate the body's surface, might appear to be capable only of treating the physical. It is not obvious to those with no knowledge of acupuncture how this physical needle placed in the body can relieve a patient's depression or soothe his emotional distress. The ancient Chinese had no trouble in understanding this, for they saw all things, and with them mankind, each as being a tiny manifestation of the Dao, the wholeness of all things, and therefore each person as potentially a complete whole in which body and soul merge together and must be treated together. A needle inserted in the body must affect the soul, just as the soul's distresses must affect the body.

There is, of course, something which we can call the health of the body, as distinct from the health of the mind or of the spirit, but the relationship between these different levels of health is always close. They cannot be treated in isolation, by sending our soul, as it were, to church and our body to hospital. The soul accompanies the body on its journey to hospital, as the body accompanies the soul to its place of spiritual repose. It is when we ignore this fact that so much unnecessary suffering is caused to those who are sick.

Once having acquired the capacity to override some of the natural conditions of life, as the human has, we have in part freed ourselves from the restrictions of our physical life. We have learnt that we can, to some extent, control nature, become her master. But we have done so at considerable cost. We have sacrificed the certainties of life lived in harmony with natural forces for the uncertainties of a world in which our ability to fashion our environment places us at odds with the smooth flow of the natural world into which we are born.

Once the body has been so effectively alienated from its surroundings as we have alienated it in the Western world, it is difficult to see how we can see nature other than as some dangerous force from whose incursions we must protect ourselves. We then live on a battleground on which man and nature appear to wage lifelong war. This is, after all, how the Western medical world views illness. But is not the truth quite other? If the universe is one, inextricably bound to itself in some great ball of energy, must not nature and man, too, be one? Acupuncture has no problem in reconciling what to the Western mind has apparently become so large a divide, for it knows that nature only works against man when man works against nature. It is we who set up the patterns of hostility, overriding nature's demands to be treated with respect. It accepts unquestioningly, indeed takes as the very heart of its practice, that nature knows what she is doing, has always known it, and that nature must thus generally be seen as a power for good.

Such, indeed, is the strength of nature's pull towards health and balance that it needs considerable force exerted against it to tilt us in the direction of ill-health and imbalance. Only repeated knocks and continuous pressure can override our natural tendency to walk upright in health through life, and the life of man, so different now from a life lived in harmony with his surroundings, provides all too many openings for such imbalances to creep in.

Traditional forms of medicine, including acupuncture, base their treatment on a belief in patients' own capacity to heal themselves. In acupuncture, the needle is used, not to inject foreign substances into the body, as with the hypodermic, but to stimulate a person's own healing mechanisms. The acupuncturist's needle, so subtle and unintrusive in its manipulations compared with its counterpart in Western medicine, is an appropriate instrument to undertake the tiny adjustments to the flow of energy through the body which are all that this energy tolerates if it is not to be disturbed and overwhelmed. The needle does not force, it extols. When used with skill, its interventions enable the energies which imbalance has blocked to flow smoothly once more within their channels as nature intends.

The elements at work

Chinese philosophy, as we have seen, has developed its own terms for describing the relentless movement of all things in the cosmos through space and time, their endless ebb and flow. It sees this cyclical movement as being the product of different phases of transformation, which we call the five elements. In each one of us, these elements are life itself poured into its physical collecting-point, our body.

In five element acupuncture we speak the symbolic language of the five elements. Symbols are a way of grasping the ungraspable, of describing the indescribable. They are a convenient and necessary abbreviation, a shorthand for the infinite. We use them for everyday communication as we speak and as we read, and in acupuncture we use them to describe those energies which give us life. The elements are symbols of all things in the process of development. This is a subtle language, profound enough to describe both delicate nuance and stark contrast, and, like all profound truths, dazzling in its simplicity, for it provides a symbolic framework embracing the dynamic concept of all life in the course of its endless transformation.

And now we need to translate what can be seen as abstract philosophical concepts into a language we can understand from everyday life by looking at one very practical example of their cyclical influence upon us, that known as jet lag. In acupuncture terms, it is quite obvious that we will suffer if we override our body's natural rhythms by wrenching ourselves from one time, season and place on this planet to another. We recognize that this must put a particular strain upon the elements and their organs within us, since these form connecting points between ourselves and what lies outside us, acting as messengers to and from the cosmos in which we are embedded.

Our organs respond to the stimuli from the different seasons and times of day upon them, and thus become confused by air travel, sending out signals of their distress which result in the unpleasant effects we call jet lag. When we fly from one time zone to another, we are in effect outrunning the sun. Our journeys bring us dawn when our bodies yearn for dusk, or winter when we have grown used to blazing summer. And then we hardly give ourselves time to adjust to these differences in time of day, season or climate before we are rattled out of any new-found equilibrium by our return flight back from summer to winter or from night to day. For this reason alone, is it little wonder that modern man and woman often fall sick? Little wonder, too, that the judgement of jet-lagged politicians must always be suspect.

Here we see evidence that the energies which feed us are influenced by those which feed nature around us. To the Chinese this was a self-evident corollary of their understanding of the oneness of all things. They understood that the energy in nature which brings to it its spring at the same time feeds our bodies through the intermediary of one of the five elements, that known as the Wood element, and through this creates and sustains the organs of the body we know of as the liver and the gallbladder. These in turn rule over specific functions which control the way our ligaments and tendons move as well as that part of our emotional energy which is associated with the desire to get things moving. By extension this has come to associate the Wood element, and thus the functions of liver and gallbladder, with those forceful expressions of our emotions we can bring under the umbrella of the word anger.

Similarly, as we shall see in greater detail later on in this book, the Fire element is our summertime, the Earth element our harvest time, the Metal element our autumn and the Water element our winter. Each provides the energy which creates specific organs of the body, and each has a similar specific function to perform within us as the different seasons perform in nature, each in turn doing what it has to do before passing on its work to the next element in what, in health, is a smooth transfer of energy in a continuous cycle around the body. In ill-health, this flow becomes disrupted, as one or other element weakens and fails to carry out its tasks properly.

When we pass from one time zone, season or climate to another, one or other, or all, of the elements within us will be forced either to abandon or accelerate what it is there to do. If we move from spring to summer in a day, the Wood element's liver and gall bladder happily going about their business of bringing spring to our lives have suddenly to stop what they are doing and hand over to the element of summer, the Fire element, whose organs, the heart and small intestine, are called upon to beam their summer warmth upon us without warning. No wonder, with such chaos within us, and such jumbled messages passing between nature outside and our organs, that we feel tired and dissociated when we have taken a long flight.

The idea that we are affected by seasonal fluctuations in this way is relatively new to the West, and has only recently been granted a brief mention in medical textbooks under the name Seasonal Affective Disorder. This lack of understanding of how each of us is influenced by what is outside us can be accounted for in part by the absence of any coherent connecting link in Western thought between living creatures and the environment in which they live. If there were a greater understanding of our immersion within the greater cosmos outside, would we not include in every hospital by far the most potentially healing of all environments, a beautiful garden, with birds singing and a waterfall flowing? Would we not also make sure that we surrounded the ill with smiling, loving faces to nurture that deepest part of them, their soul?

We seem in the West to concentrate our attention upon trying to counter influences upon us from outside which are predominantly harmful, such as the effects of pollution or food poisoning. Here nature becomes a hostile force creating illness. The concept of a healthy, life-giving and life-enhancing communion between man and nature which nourishes both has up to now been alien to Western thought, and is only moving a little more centre-stage as we begin to see the visible effects of ignoring such interactions (global warming, pollution of the environment) where what damages one part of this nature/mankind equation must damage the other, and what is health for one is health for the other.

In Chinese medical thought, man is embedded in nature, nourished by nature, at one with nature. The energies which feed nature outside, making the flowers grow and the birds sing, continue their flow within us, making our hearts sing and our bodies flourish. We can access these energies, miraculously I still feel after all these years in acupuncture, through a needle placed in an acupuncture point lying along one of the meridians shown on the chart. In so doing, if we select the correct point at the correct time and for the correct purpose, the impulse imparted to the acupuncture point by the insertion of the needle gives a tiny jolt, moving our patient the slightest bit away from ill-health and nudging him towards health. This is what enables us to realign a patient's energies to counteract the dislocation caused by air travel.

This constant interaction between nature and ourselves, as the daily and seasonal cycle feed the energies of the elements, is regarded by the ancient Chinese as being as necessary a source of nourishment as the intake of air and food we all recognize as being essential to our survival. This tight interlocking of ourselves with the natural world symbolizes a growing out, a budding forth, of our being towards the cosmic forces which swirl around us, as every cell of body and soul responds to the swirling tides and fluctuating energies of the natural world beyond us.

When, then, we look at the individual sources of energy within the human being we call the elements, we must keep always in mind a picture of them which embeds them in the whole. And each of us, apparently standing, in our own patch of sunlight, must always be seen as being as tightly clasped to nature's bosom as is a tree rooted to the ground. Because we are so used to seeing all living creatures moving around, we may tend to forget how tightly we, no less than any tree, are enmeshed, cell by cell, with all that is around us, unless we are acupuncturists, or other practitioners of disciplines based upon the movement of energies, who use these connections as the foundation of their practice.

CHAPTER 2

OUR TRUE SHAPE

The universe condenses itself at one point in space and time to form the tiny unit of life which is to become a human being, bestowing upon us sufficient energy to last the span of whatever lifetime we have been allotted. And when our life has run its course, has completed the purpose of its creation, we discard our identity in the dissolution of death to merge once more with all that is. Life is an infinite process of renewal, a progression from life to death and back again.

That great breath of life which the universe breathes into us at the moment of our creation bears within it our individual mark. We each flow to a unique shape. On the face of the earth there is, has been and will be nobody else who is exactly like me. I am the only one of my kind, as we all are. This makes me feel both lonely and proud. I am the bearer of a unique burden. Whether I like it or not, I cannot escape the fact that I am uniquely myself, and as such to be treated with infinite care and compassion.

And I owe myself profound respect. If the like of me will never be seen again then I must ensure that the span of my life, tiny though it might appear when measured against eternity, should be as fruitful and true to itself as I can make it. I must learn to respect the contours of my particular shape, for this is the only shape I will ever have, and to distort or conceal it is a denial of that inner core of me, my unique self. I owe it to myself to be myself.

The contours of that unique shape to which we all flow are outlined and filled in by the details of our life. It is a dynamic shape, moulding itself around the pressures which life puts upon it, swelling and diminishing, bulging and collapsing as it withstands these pressures or succumbs to their weight. It is in eternal tension with the outside world, and has endlessly to balance what is wanted of it against what is rightful for it, a tension which can be creative or negative, leading either to our growth or to our diminution. If life presses too hard upon us, and we have not the strength to resist this pressure, it will deform us, the beautiful shape we have been born with gradually distorting itself, because it has not learnt to guard its contours carefully.

Our true shape, which is bestowed upon us as a gift for life, can be distorted, concealed or denied, but cannot, except by death, be obliterated. It makes its presence felt through the energies flowing within us, those energies which make our minds think, our bodies move and our souls feel. The Chinese discovered that the very shape of our bodies is defined and delineated by these energies. Like sap flowing through branches, these breathed life into our bodies, and, like sap leaving the branches, they brought death in their wake when their flow was impeded. This life-shaping energy endlessly circled through us according to the rhythm of the five elements, five fairy godmothers each offering in turn its special gift.

Our body is the physical receptacle for this flow of energy, but it is home not only to our physical being but to our thoughts and passions. It provides shelter for our physical energy, for those much profounder energies which breathe life into our mind and for the most profound of all, those which animate our soul. Whatever touches our body touches our soul. Whatever joys our body experiences render our soul joyful. Whatever blows our body receives also hammer our soul. We are given this coarse, crude, often malfunctioning container, the body, to shelter this exquisite, pure and gentle soul, at a stroke creating the background for that great lifelong struggle between body and soul, between those forces which tie our bodies down to the earth and those which strive to soar upwards to the heavens. This is a conflict which neither body nor soul can win. Our bodies can never rid themselves of that which breathes life into them. Our souls cannot escape from the confines of the physical body until that moment of death.

How then do we know what our true shape is, and learn to defend its contours? It is always a gradual process. We have been given our outline, deep within which glimmers that untarnishable diamond, our unique and precious soul, but this outline can easily become misshapen by what the world does to us. If we live with unwise parents in an unwise world, the tiny, growing, budding thing which is us as a child may not be nurtured or loved or supported or watched over as it should be. We cannot blame others for this. If they, too, have in their turn suffered from neglect, how can they know what it is to give succour and shelter to their child's soul and body? As the years go by, our tiny soul, which was placed inside the perfect circle of our first cell, may grow outwards with bumps and dents upon it, until, by the time it is fully adult, its outlines may become jagged and tattered. The cruel, harsh edges which distort us now catch at the world and its people as they flow around and past us, pulling further out of shape both us and all who touch us.

Fruitful interplay between us and the world outside is always necessary. We grow to recognize who we are by learning to develop our own responses to outside pressures, gradually taking over this role from those into whose protective arms we are placed when we are born. Some of us never fully accept this role, refusing to take on responsibility for ourselves, and others of us will be so anxious to rid ourselves of this protection that we deny it the right to teach us anything, cutting ourselves free before we are ready. In either case, the gradual emergence of us as mature people will become impeded. Those weeds of the past will trail in our wake, tugging at us, pulling us down and sometimes drowning us.

Our shape in full maturity should flow in a beautiful circle around and past all we encounter, undistorting and undistortable, its contours so smoothed by the creative interaction with life that no jagged edges tear and pull off-balance. Such a smooth circle will eventually become strong enough to withstand the onslaughts from all those cruel hooks with which others, in their immaturity and distress, may in their turn approach us. And one of the most heartening things about such a picture is that as our contours flow ever more smoothly, so the shape of those who come into contact with us begins to lose some of its sharp and hurting edges. We have the ability to tear each other to pieces in our imbalance, or to complete each other in our balance, for our refusal to allow others to distort us strengthens and firmly delineates our boundaries, helping others to discover their own.

We have each been assigned a certain shape, each our own space within which to act out our lives. It surrounds and encircles us, and we can never escape from it. Our view of the world outside is through and from within this space. This precious place has to be guarded jealously from encroachment. Nobody has a right to enter it without our permission, and we must respect the spaces of all we encounter. We enter in awed and hushed tones into any sacred place, and each soul is a sacred place to be held in trust by us for the span of our lifetime. That precious energy which breathes life into us is the watchful guardian of our true shape. The pathways of energy which acupuncture recognizes flow in an endless circle around our body, constantly redressing the distortions of life by giving us the strength to develop firm boundaries of our own. Just as the strength of sap within a leaf will define the shape of that leaf, so we are shaped by the strength of the energy flowing within us.

If the currents of our energy start to falter, far from assisting us they start instead to impede us. It is as though we flow against the tide of ourselves. Our true self becomes increasingly untrue to itself, denying itself. And we deny ourselves at our peril, squeezing ourselves into something more closely resembling a straitjacket than the beautiful flowing circle we should all be. Our increasing refusal to see ourselves for what we are leads us away from a full life to a kind of half-life lived among shadows, or, if our attempts to deny ourselves become overwhelming, to the gradual denial of life itself.

When the pressures of life prove too strong for us to withstand, our energy loses some of its ability to support us. Its flow falters. As its strengthening hold upon us weakens, our body and soul weaken with it, and as they weaken, they become ailing, and disease takes hold. It matters little whether this is disease of the body or of the soul, for disease of the body must eventually affect the soul, and disease of the soul cannot leave the body untouched. The flow of energy is one, uniting body to soul and soul to body.

If, like some rosebud disguised as an acorn, or a sparrow in the guise of a hawk, we fail to be who we are by pretending to be who we are not, we will do all we can to prevent our cover being blown, for this disguise is so well embedded in our life that removing it must inevitably lead to profound and often uncomfortable changes. It cannot be otherwise. If we have so far lived as oak-like a life as possible, it is not easy to accept that the graceful, poetic rosebush is where we belong, and yet we have to be prepared to make such radical adjustments as we grow towards our true shape. If we do not, we will find our acorn-disguise sitting ever more uneasily upon us, as the natural shape we are born with increasingly exerts its pressure to be allowed to be itself.

The tensions of trying to shape our lives according to others' demands rather than our own needs will reveal themselves in clear guise within us. It seems that, so intent are we on ensuring that our mask remains on, we fail to notice that its faithful shadow, our true self, has taken the opportunity to slip away unnoticed to signal its distress behind our back. It is as though one hand masks us, while the other unmasks us. We apparently wish to hide our distresses and pains, and yet we reveal them in all we do.

When our life flows with us, it flows smoothly, unafraid of the light of day. Then we are not ashamed proudly to declare 'This is who I am.' But if we hide our true shape, it forces itself secretly to our attention. Shadows of unrest flit across our faces, hide in our voices, conceal themselves in our emotions, silent cries of distress. Acupuncturists are trained to hear these cries and trace them to their source. The cries are often faint, and come from the far distance, well hidden by all our defences, but with time, patience and skill we gradually find our way to that source. We are interpreters. We use the dictionary of the elements to interpret the language of distress our patients talk.

But those cries may go unheeded for the span of our life. The negative shadows sweeping over us can gradually become so dense and impenetrable that we become hidden within them. We lose ourselves within ourselves, and never find ourselves again. The path through such deep mists must lead permanently away from that joyous journey of self-discovery. It is as though the one thing which we were born to say, that one triumphant declaration, 'I am who I am', is stifled on our lips. We die not knowing who we are. We have denied our soul its moment of glorious self-assertion.

The guardian element

We must now start to translate into the language of acupuncture the challenges each of us is faced with as we struggle to maintain our right to be ourselves.

What neither the Da Vinci cartoon nor the acupuncture chart from Chapter 1 can show, for they are not sufficiently multi-dimensional, is how the image of a human being which they depict develops through time and space. To move us forward from birth to death, and from this place to the next, the wheel into which we fit must turn, the circle transform itself into a spiral. Each cycle of life, each moment in time, as it turns back on itself to become the next cycle, the next moment, does so at a slightly different level, just as ring is added to ring to form the trunk of a tree. Things never remain the same. Each spring is a new spring unlike any that has gone before, finding the trees upon which it sprouts its buds a little taller or more withered, these buds endowed with a little more or less vitality. Within us, too, time works away, each moment finding us a little changed from the moment which precedes it, at each stage of our life giving us the potential to change and develop.

Unlike the drawing or the chart, which are fixed eternally at one moment of this cycling, our life is therefore a constant dynamic of change and development, as the elements, the symbolic representation of the wheeling of time, add each a slightly different focus to what has gone before. Nor can the drawing or chart show the human being as the unique individuals we know ourselves to be. They sketch us in the most universal, and thus impersonal terms, offering a meagre, empty outline of ourselves, all our individual characteristics etched out to reveal only a symbolic illustration, just as a map of a town cannot show the teeming lives of its inhabitants. Designed to encapsulate all of mankind in one single series of outlines, what these two-dimensional, static illustrations cannot show is what breathes life into us, fills us out, makes us who we are, lights each of us from within with our own individual spark, that tiny flame piercing the darkness of cosmic night which is an individual life. It is this flame, burning sometimes brightly in health, sometimes flickering or fading in ill-health, which lights this book. And it is my task as acupuncturist to help that flame burn steadily and truly in each of my patients.

Deep within all of us, however securely we attempt to absorb ourselves into the company of others, like drops of water on to blotting paper, there pulses the individual soul, with its own needs and thoughts and desires and beliefs, and with its own path of self-development beckoning it to detach itself from its fellows and move us into the often frightening light of our own self-expression. We slip each into a solitary life at birth, as though stepping into a garment prepared especially for us.

The attributes we have in common with one another, which define our membership of a particular species, though announcing their common origin, on close analysis yield signs of awesome uniqueness. The forces of the universe which pour their energies into us to create us are transformed within each of us into something that is so unique that a drop of blood or a single hair will differentiate us from anyone else who has ever existed, exists now or will exist. Each of us can thus be seen as a tiny, but unique, emanation of the Dao, formed of the fusion of yin/yang and the five elements.

To the ancient Chinese these forms of yin/yang and the five elements, creating as they do all things, also necessarily create the individual characteristics which make you in many ways unlike me, despite the two of us having a myriad of characteristics our species has in common. In their ancient wisdom they built up a comprehensive spread of individual features attributing specific qualities out of the complete range of human qualities to each one of us, and offering us their own satisfying explanations for the human diversity we all manifest. This they translated into the language of the elements, seeing our individuality as a product of the elements' unique signatures upon us.

The energies of the elements flow through all things, creating all things, and they flow through each of us in a unique way, shaping us, in body and soul, according to a unique template, a stamp all our own which is the elemental equivalent of our individual genetic inheritance. There is much discussion as to the nature of this imprint. Some say that it is the vicissitudes of life which stamp it upon us, others believe, as I do, that, like our genetic makeup, it is there in our first cell and stays constant within us throughout our life. It makes us who we are.

The elements flow to a rhythm within us, their interplay determining who we are. Much as a painter can never put together an assembly of colours in exactly the same combination of pigments each time he mixes his paints, so the combination of elements which goes to make up our individual colour cannot be replicated elsewhere. Upon all of us they lay a hand of blessing, but one in particular has been selected as our special guardian to watch over and protect us, singling us out to bestow upon us the responsibility of our own individuality. With this element we each have a unique relationship. I call it our guardian element.

In everything we do and everything we are we shout out our allegiance to this element. It puts its special seal upon us, and we bear its distinguishing mark printed upon face and body and emotion, no more to be altered than can the colour of our eyes or the size of our bones. We are who we are because we have received the gift of its patronage. So profound is the influence of this element, so all-pervasive is its mark upon us, that it lays a visible, palpable, audible signature upon us, writ large on our bodies, to be interpreted by eye and ear, and by touch and smell. It reveals itself by giving a specific colour to our face (not to be confused with racial colouring), a specific sound to our voice and a specific smell upon our body.

My voice, for example, is not just a disembodied voice. It emerges from deep within me, and expresses who I am and what I am and how I am at any moment in time. It is the product of the unique interaction of the elements' work within me, and is sufficiently distinct that my voice print can now open doors for me which will remain closed to any other voice. Similarly my smell and the colour upon my skin are unique to me and cannot be replicated elsewhere. They therefore offer unique diagnostic information if interpreted correctly.

Our element also endows us with a specific emotional orientation to our life which throws a patina of its own over all that we do. This emotional filter colours the way we see things, the way we respond to things, the way we move. It will affect the way we express ourselves in words as well as in action, and the way we perceive things. Some of us may find a person reassuring whom others feel threatened by. Some are happier moving within touching range of people, whilst others dislike physical contact and demand space around them. There are quick movers amongst us, and those who move ponderously, as there are fluent talkers and those with little words.

We come into the world blessed with the special gift of one of the elements, and with this gift, the potential for using it either wisely or unwisely, of choosing to live within the shadows of its dark side rather than in its bright sunlight. And thus each of our five guardians comes with its own dark companion, its Mephistopheles dogging its every footstep. Such positive, creative forces trail in their wake negative, destructive forces. Like everything else, an element can become a force for good or a force for ill. It can show us the way forward or bring us to a halt.

Each of us in our uniqueness can thus be seen as reflecting reality from a slightly different angle. The tilt of that angle, its particular emphasis, is the product of the unique balance of the elements within us, and of the dominant position of one element. It forms the hub of the wheel of our life around which the other elements circle. All the other elements within us feel stronger if it is strong, grow weaker as it weakens. It is the focal point of each of our lives, dictating by its health or ill-health whether or not we will remain balanced within ourselves. It forms the core of our individuality. To those trained to detect the marks of the elements upon us, we appear each as a physical manifestation of the presence and power of this element within us.

Our response to the stresses of life, as they act themselves out upon the elements, is therefore no haphazard process. The characteristics of our guardian element, determining as they do all that affects our life, will also determine the nature of our individual response to the difficulties we encounter. The way in which we fall ill will thus be as much influenced by our guardian element as will the way in which we fall in love, the jobs we do, the way we walk and talk and what we find funny or sad. Every facet of an individual life will be orientated towards that one segment of the complete cycle of the elements represented by this element.

The closest we come in the West to determining individual traits in a comparable way to this is when we categorize people as belonging to certain character types. The ancient medical concept of the humours, consigned long ago to gather dust on the shelves of medical libraries, also approaches this concept of the guardian element. Such systems of medicine, and others around the world, predominantly in the East, such as the Indian and Japanese systems, all share a common belief that we shape our illnesses, that the type of person we are is a factor in the way in which we succumb to disease, and that we have a constitutional predisposition to certain imbalances.

Our element imposes its own obligations upon us, for to live our life in balance requires us to live that life in tune with our element's demands. When we run true to its needs, we find a direction to our life which is fruitful. Many of my patients will tell me things like, 'I feel more myself now than I have ever felt', or, 'I know now who I am.' When we run counter to our element's needs, we lose our way, as though the undergrowth closes over the path we should take. Then our element turns from guardian into avenging angel, exacting revenge from us in the shape of ill-health and distress. To that extent we are not free, much as we are not free to choose when we are born, to which parents we are born, whether we are born poor or rich, tall or short, curly- or straight-haired.

How we view our individual destinies hinges to a large extent upon the vision we each hold about what life is about. I cannot accept that a human life can be nothing but the sum total of its inherited characteristics, determined purely by parental adequacies and inadequacies, with nothing added of some spark of individuality, giving to these characteristics something more and something different. It seems clear to me that the tiny soul, emerging untarnished from its mother's womb, brings with it into the world something uniquely its own, seen physically as its unique genetic imprint. Translated into the language of the elements, that imprint corresponds to a unique elemental imprint.

Upon no other species has such a variety of individual characteristics been bestowed as its share of cosmic bounty. The scope for diversity with which this endows humankind is thus potentially as infinite as the number of human beings born on this planet. We must each find our own explanation for the development of such highly individual qualities which characterize our species. I like to think that the impetus within us to evolve towards ever higher levels of diversification became so overriding at some point in our evolution that we were no longer able to contain within each of us the totality of characteristics which make up humankind. Our very complexity appears to have placed so great a burden upon our individual capacity to absorb the awesome range of powers the human being has developed that we might be said to have burst the bounds of what each of us can encompass within ourselves of the human condition, becoming dispersed into so many fragments of the whole.

The potential for our achievements thus appears to be pinpointed upon one segment of the whole, like a spotlight, focused upon one area of the human stage. Our specifically human characteristics appear to have been honed down until we have each become, not merely representatives of a species, but individuals owing allegiance to no type but ourselves, each of us, in effect potentially a one man/one woman species of our own, with such distinct individuality that a businessman and a poet, sharing the same generic body, can be as alien to one another as can be a butterfly to a kangaroo.

Our individual philosophy of life will dictate whether we see the high degree of human variety as being the result of a chance concatenation of genes, a random shaking of the kaleidoscope of human characteristics, or view it as the expression of a tiny purpose in the cosmic mind, endowing each of us with our own sublime significance, and making us subtly, yet clearly, unique, with the potential to offer to the stock of human endeavour our own individual contribution of a life lived badly or well. It is my belief that each of our lives is endowed with such a purpose, and this belief underlies this book. It also implicitly underlies the practice of five element acupuncture, for its treatment is directed at what it regards as the cause of all imbalance, the inability of the guardian element to maintain sufficient strength and focus to allow us to fulfil the unique aim of our life as expressed through this element.

Why does imbalance occur?

If we posit a natural order, as the ancient Chinese did, how and why do the imbalances and disturbances all humankind is heir to occur? There is no hint of disharmony in Leonardo's drawing or the acupuncture chart from Chapter 1. The wheel which the body forms could, we feel, rotate endlessly unto infinity in its perfect symmetry of movement. A sense of human contentment sits easily within such a picture of harmony, but it appears not to accommodate the frequent episodes of illness and unhappiness which punctuate our lives. What is it in the human condition that allows for such a level of imbalance?

Perhaps one explanation among many possible ones can be found in our very uniqueness, for we are the most complex creatures on God's earth, our evolutionary development having endowed us with manifold characteristics so far denied any

other species of which we are aware, and it is by no means easy
for all these complex structures and functions to maintain their
balance. This very complexity therefore brings complications of
all kinds in its wake which no other creature appears to suffer
to the same degree.

If we see the body as a delicate mechanism within which
different energies constantly balance themselves against one
another to maintain life, it is clear that the chances of this
mechanism malfunctioning will increase the more highly
evolved it becomes and the greater the stresses to which it
is subjected. The very high level of human complexity, our
intricate brain, our deep capacity for an emotional life, our
highly evolved body, all packaged so neatly within an animal
space of no more than average size, have not made it easy for
such a complicated mechanism to function as it should all the
time. The endless readjustments and fine tuning required of the
human body and soul, whilst giving to them an impressively
wide range of functions, also bring with them the need for
constant running repairs to their intricate mechanisms. All
this makes the possibility of breakdown so much more likely.
The stresses these powerful forces place upon us, with their
insatiable demand for satisfaction and fulfilment, create a
specifically human dilemma.

Physical stresses, arising from the tension between the needs
of our body and the environment's greater or lesser capacity
for fulfilling them, are factors we have in common with all
forms of life, from the plant to the animal. But, in the human
being, to these must be added the increasing stresses created
by those deeper, inner forces within us. Indeed, it could be
said that the need to satisfy our physical demands has slowly
been superseded by that of satisfying our inner demands. We
have gradually turned our efforts inwards, and in this process
of internalization the focal point of our life has shifted from
attention to its external aspects, the gaining of food, the
provision of shelter, to increased concentration upon feeding

our inner being, the gaining of knowledge, the achievement of emotional stability or the creation of artistic achievement. We can microwave in five minutes what it took our primitive ancestor a year to produce, and all this and much other saved time has allowed us the luxury of deepening our thoughts. We now have the option of reading a book or going to a film, where this ancestor of ours knew no such marvels of abstract thought, and had to be content, of a dark and cheerless evening, with sleep.

The development of such a high degree of complexity appears to have been bought at the expense of the cohesion of the whole, bringing with it abundant scope for conflict and discord. For in developing the highly individual characteristics all human beings show we may potentially have had to forfeit some of our overall balance. And it is our guardian element which pays the price for playing such an important role, if its energy proves insufficient to bear the weight of all that is demanded of it. This element's hold on balance is thus always to some extent precarious because of the primacy of its position, its very importance making it vulnerable. If we put all our eggs in one elemental basket, as it were, that basket is likely to feel the strain. Our element is thus both our greatest blessing, endowing us with all the gifts which make of us the unique human being each of us is, and, potentially, also our greatest curse. For if we deny ourselves the right to be who we uniquely are it is upon this element that the greatest burden will fall.

And, too, all the efforts we have made over the millennia to draw ourselves up from the primaeval slime out into the daylight have brought with them their own burdens, endowing us with that particularly human quality, which is a mixture of pride and humility, giving us on the one hand an arrogant belief in our great skills of mind and body, on the other a recognition of our deep inadequacies. It would seem that we have bought a heightened sense of awareness at the high price of the uneasy self-doubts which accompany it. Dissatisfaction and inner turmoil, the shadow-side of the gifts of self-fulfilment, are the heavy price we pay for our almost limitless potential for self-development. This is the dilemma of modern mankind, whose strivings have lifted us far beyond the limitations of our ancestors, only to expose us to the doubts and longings of a soul in search of itself.

If we look inwards, we find a world in which our inner horizons know no limits, for they open upon eternity. If we look outwards and view ourselves from far out in space, we see a perfect globe into which the millions upon millions of us neatly fit, so many ants in our ant-heap. Our ability to expand our inner and outer horizons in this way places its own pressures upon us, for the panorama they reveal is both elating and terrifying. Recognizing that we form part of a great whole, how small and insignificant yet we may feel that part now to be. It is ironic that the superimposition of the infinity of world upon world revealed by our telescopes should bestow significance upon all things by revealing their interconnectedness and yet may rob these things individually of that very significance by drowning them as tiny droplets in the great oceans of time and space. By widening our horizons to gain the greater picture we threaten our conviction of our own importance.

And thus we can choose to feel ourselves both everything or nothing, both supremely important as a crucial part of the interlocking pattern of the universe, and supremely unimportant as we are swamped by the sheer immensity of that pattern's scale. All things henceforth become gigantic in their proportions. We can no longer shelter within a universe scaled to our size. We are either dwarfed by its hugeness or ourselves made huge by the minute dimensions of the microcosmic world. Our view of ourselves in relation to the cosmos has dramatically shifted and can tilt dangerously to one side or the other. One of our difficulties is then to find our own point of equilibrium between these two extremes of mankind as nothing and mankind as everything.

And these uncertainties lead us to question the purpose of life, and to ponder upon life's mysteries. No other animal's breast heaves with such existential torments; no other species lies sleepless under the night's canopy of stars, awestruck by the deep mystery of those immense spaces. Only upon us, with our powers of concentrated introspection, has the dilemma of existence made such a devastating impact, subjecting us to such deep uncertainties. Hence such a high level of discontent. Hence such dissatisfactions, such prickings and railings at fate.

And thus at the present pinnacle of evolution we sit uneasily, jarring the harmony of the natural scene with our dissatisfactions, our inner turmoils, our griefs and pains and illnesses, where the rest of nature lives life out so unquestioningly. It could be said that, seen from a human perspective, those vast cosmic powers which order the universe have thrown, with mankind, a grain of sand into the smooth workings of nature. Little wonder, then, that we feel anxious and unsafe, prone to self-doubt and unsure of our own significance. And thus, with us, doubt enters the universe, bringing with it as its necessary companion the exhilaration of the possible, the lure of the question mark. A future pregnant with the possibilities of new horizons opens up. Querying what is before us, we refuse to accept that this world as we know it is all that there is to know. We look beneath and behind and beyond.

Here, indeed, the scene is set for a great drama of human life in which Man, sprung from nature and subject always to its laws, yet finds himself, by virtue of his unique gifts, the only species on this earth uncertain as to his place in the scheme of things. Nor can he attempt to retreat back down the evolutionary ladder to rejoin his fellow animals in their unquestioning subservience to nature, for his ability to think and alter his environment has made this impossible. He must, perforce, accept the limitations of a life in which he has forfeited the unchanging, unthinking, uncreative world of most of his forbears for a confused world where, having forced himself to stand to some extent apart from the rest of nature, his very isolation makes him vulnerable.

All other animals appear to fit happily within their allotted fate. The zebra on the plain, the ant in its ant heap, the bee in its hive, all appear, to human eyes at least, to accept their place within the cosmic order. Even the domesticated animal, endowed through contact with the human world with a few more obviously individual characteristics, will not of its own accord attempt to alter its environment or change its way of life. We, by contrast, are not content with remaining as we are. The impulse which prompted our ancestors far back in time to stand up on their hind-legs and reach out around them and to the stars above appears to find its echo in each of us, as we long for what is beyond us. We appear to have sacrificed a life lived in unquestioning harmony with the natural world for far more uncertain, but more challenging horizons.

The disturbing thing here is the scale of the human capacity for imbalance. The picture is not of the smooth flow of things, but of a difficult and often tortured climb through life. This seems to bear no resemblance at all to Leonardo's image of perfect symmetry. Rather, it takes on a much more distorted shape, with jagged edges and no centre to hold all together. And this creates for each of us an exhilarating but potentially troubled life.

Given the scale of all these pressures upon us, little wonder that we grasp eagerly for whatever support we can find to guide us through such often frightening wildernesses. And drive us, too, to seek help from amongst the myriad of therapies now available to enable us, however temporarily, to share and we hope ultimately to shed some of this load, amongst them acupuncture.

What is balance?

Before we look closely at each element in its manifold manifestations within each one of us, we need to look at what we call health, and what we consider to be a healthy and balanced state. And we can feel ourselves to be out of balance in soul as well as in body, the ills of the former scoring often more deeply into us than those of the body. In this book we will be talking of the widest range of health, that which covers all aspects of human life.

It could be said that health is not something we bother our heads about much when we are healthy. It is a form of well-being which the healthy take for granted but which the unhealthy long for and clamour vigorously for from the wide range of therapies on offer. One definition of health is to see it as a state of being in which we successfully balance different needs within us. Physically, for example, this would be seen as the needs of the heart being balanced against the needs of the lungs. Mentally, the needs of our work must be balanced against the need for quiet and repose, and spiritually, the needs of our deepest being, for love and passion and profound thoughts, must be weighed against the need for contented living. Ill-health is when these creative tensions topple over into destructive phases.

Within this equation of health-creative tension/ill-health-destructive tension lies a further, more elusive factor, which adds a more complex layer to human struggles. We know that different people are subject to different sorts of tension. The thrusting businessman will find competitive tensions with business partners stimulating, whilst another will find such abrasiveness disturbing. One of us will deal happily with another's anger, whilst that same anger may crush someone else. These differences arise from our individual responses, and these in turn are shaped by what makes us who we are, by the uniqueness of our being.

Every part of us has its own way of revealing its distress. In the body, it will be by the experiencing of pain, the appearance of physical changes, such as lumps, discolouration or raised temperature, by structural changes, such as tightening of the ligaments or bowing of the bones. In the mind, it can express itself by unquiet thoughts, uncertainties, obsessive worries. The soul's distresses can appear as emotional imbalance, uncontrolled anger or deep sadness, the inability to express love or warmth, feelings of despair and desolation, a profound questioning of whether our life has purpose.

Each of these manifold signs of distress is a pointer to what acupuncturists call an imbalance in energy. The aim of all treatment is to trace to their source the patterns of imbalance woven by the distress signals sent out by the elements. Everything that has happened to a patient on that journey towards imbalance is relevant, however apparently insignificant the details, for all imbalances are seen as having a cause. Pain and discomfort do not appear out of the blue, but are the result of some dislocation to the smooth flow of energy connecting element to element. Imbalances in energy are seen as revealing themselves initially, not in the dramatic appearance of a malignant tumour, the trembling limbs of an MS patient or a mental breakdown, but as tiny shifts in energy, in a hint of snappiness where we were previously good-tempered, in an inability to tolerate certain foods, in a change in the colours we like wearing, in an ache in the knee or a twinge in the back.

If every part of us is seen as connected to every other part, it is obvious that when any of these parts falls sick, this sickness will reflect itself in some way throughout the whole, much like an infection from a small cut on the finger will cause a fever to spread throughout our body. Even the slightest knock to any part of the energy system will reverberate around the body, setting off a chain-reaction from element to element and from organ to organ.

Though ills may manifest themselves at one or other level of body or soul, each may well cause after-shocks at the other levels, initially possibly slight, and then with increasing time deeper, until with severe ill-health all the layers of our being are affected. We have mechanisms to prevent flooding of the system. We can suppress ills of the body with painkilling drugs and ills of the soul with anti-depressants, but only for a time, and then the disturbance surfaces again, often in a more troubling way. We can deny we are overtired (ills of the body) and keep ourselves at our desk with caffeine or alcohol, but eventually such denial is useless. We become depressed and irritable. We cannot sleep when we eventually get to bed, and sleeping-pills gradually lose their effect. Finally, we have to seek greater help than that offered by the pharmacist or the pub.

Let us imagine we are walking along arm-in-arm with our beloved, our souls at peace, our mind pondering gently on where we will go for a meal. What happens then if, walking along in this bubble of contentment, we stub our toe on the pavement? Immediately the feeling of peace is shattered, the bubble bursts. Suddenly this contented body of ours is aware of sharp pain, our being is plucked out of its contentment and we will be unable to settle back into our happy state until the pain has subsided. If we have broken our toe, the peace will vanish for some time.

The same disturbance will happen if during this peaceful walk our mobile phone rings and somebody tells us of trouble at the office, or if our partner suddenly talks about being unhappy in our relationship. Here the disruption is at the level, first, of the mind, then of the soul, as the words being spoken are deciphered and then their meaning interpreted. To a lesser or greater extent, disruptions of any kind threaten our state of balance, attacking either body or soul, and requiring much attention and hard work from us to bring them back under control so that metaphorically we can continue to walk peacefully along the path of our life.

A serious physical ailment, such as a heart attack or cancer, will immediately affect our mind and spirit ('Am I going to die?', 'Who will look after my children?', 'How will I cope with the pain?'), just as a serious emotional problem will give us migraines or stomach ulcers. A stubbed or broken toe will mend, and the degree of inconvenience it brings with it, such as difficulty in walking or driving the car, will vary depending on how much we need to walk or drive a car. Worries at the office may be harder to dispel, and troubles in our relationship will disturb us the most. Here we see the different levels of our being revealing the degree of their relative importance to us. We can manage surprisingly well initially if it is only our body which is under stress. The moment the deeper levels of our being are involved, the deeper the discontent will be driven inside us, to the extent that we may eventually be unable to find ways of dealing with it without the help of outside intervention.

When we are healthy, the energy feeding the elements will supply what the body and soul need to maintain their state of health. In balance, we will arrange our lives in such a way that the needs of our guardian element are met so that it is able to fulfil its function adequately. There will be neither too much nor too little of any particular form of energy, but just the right amount to maintain balance. But under stress the elements will threaten the balance which they are there to provide. Where they should be fulfilling our needs, they may start instead to undermine us, refusing to give where they are needed or taking where they should be giving. This happens, for example, when we fall ill with pneumonia, and our lungs, struggling to breathe, are unable to supply oxygen to the other parts of the body as they should. Our balance can only be maintained if there is unselfish co-operation between the energies feeding us, much as, in the physical body, the heart and lungs must be prepared to pump blood or oxygen to wherever they are needed. The different energies must therefore perform unselfishly for the good of the whole.

But when we are out of balance, our perceptions of what is right for us will become distorted, encouraging us to do that which tends to throw us further off-balance. And any stresses which an element is unable to absorb become a destructive force if left unchecked, reducing that element's capacity to function as it should. As one element weakens, greater demands are placed upon the others to support it, and they, in turn, will eventually also suffer. With time, unless something is done to counter this, the whole energy structure of body and soul will be undermined, opening up gaps where disease can all too easily creep in.

Just as rifts and cracks in the surface of the earth may herald the approach of an earthquake seething unseen below our feet, so must we learn to regard the rifts and cracks in our health, those headaches and sleepless nights, joint pains and fevers, as advance warnings of trouble ahead to which we must pay heed if the whole edifice of our health is not to be undermined. And yet it is surprising how much we take the very existence of illness as a permanent accompaniment to our lives so for granted that it occasions little notice when we fall prey to its different manifestations. And we appear to accept equally without surprise those times when we are miserable or depressed. How rare, we may think, are the days when we wake totally refreshed and content with our lot. And if we do, how many of such days find us then going to bed with that contentment undermined rather than reinforced?

When we are in tune with ourselves and the universe we are healthy and contented. Nothing within us jars to draw us away from this feeling of well-being. In some ways we are unaware of ourselves. The dividing-line between inside and outside seems to have disappeared and we are at one with things. And yet it requires little for that balance to be upset, the merest withholding of breath, absence of the right food constituent or a friend's frown, and the delicate regulatory functions inside us grow confused and unable to respond appropriately. We need only remind ourselves here of what happens if we sit in a draught or begin to feel hungry, and how quickly we feel impelled to take action to make ourselves feel comfortable again.

If we do not, imbalance and disharmony creep in. The scales tilt away from the level which is our state of equilibrium towards a condition of too much or too little. As one thing slides out of balance, it draws another with it, increasing the disequilibrium to a point where harmony can no longer be restored. Eventually, if unchecked, this becomes the onset of what we call illness, the point at which our mechanisms for re-establishing our own balance have succumbed to overwhelming pressure from forces operating against our welfare. We begin to be at war with ourselves, in our misery unable to distinguish appropriate from inappropriate functioning.

And yet we will retain a memory of health and balance which dims beyond recall only when we become too ill and have passed beyond the point of recovery. And it is this memory of healthy times past which comes to acupuncture's aid when the first treatment is given and the first needle inserted. For the body craves health, as a fish craves water and a bird its life on the wing. We are at ease within it, and seek it desperately when we have lost it. We take it for granted when we possess it, a thing almost invisible in its presence, and yet its absence dominates our life, allowing us room for little else but our craving to get better.

For it appears that all things in the universe bear deep within themselves a striving towards wholeness. We need only think of all those jagged fragments of matter torn apart in explosions far out in cosmic time and space floating out there in the ether. However broken their edges, they slowly succumb to the force of cosmic laws, eventually becoming smoothed into a perfect circle, each again a small reflection of cosmic wholeness. And then what a thing of beauty these broken pieces of matter become, torn apart in some primaeval explosion, but, like the once fragmented earth, transformed into a globe of awesome harmony.

All this activity on a cosmic scale is the work of the elements, as they strive to draw things back into a whole again. On a human scale, they welcome the needle in this work as it gently coaxes the elements' constant search for wholeness. I can find no other explanation for the extraordinary feelings of well-being acupuncture treatment can evoke in us, as, with a sigh of relief, we become more ourselves.

Has imbalance a function?

What relevance to acupuncture have such ponderings, and why does the acupuncturist need to think of such things? It is because we are concerned with human suffering. The whole range of human distress, whether physical or at a deeper level within us, is the field on which acupuncture works. The impetus which forces us to seek help of others, and hence of an acupuncturist, always comes from some spur of pain. And thus the acupuncturist must learn to place human suffering and human joy in some context. Faced with the despairs, unhappinesses and physical ailments brought to us by our patients, we must work towards our own understanding of the significance of all this suffering. At every turn we are forced to confront questions relating to human destiny and the purpose of human striving.

If we are to help someone back to health, we must learn to distinguish between what is healthy and what is unhealthy for that particular patient. Our work is done in the gap between these two states, as we try to transform the unbalanced into the balanced. Many factors, personal and social, contribute to our assessment of the level of imbalance we ourselves or others are suffering, and different cultures find a lesser or greater degree of discomfort more acceptable than others. The sailor in Nelson's navy prided himself on not allowing a single sound to escape as his limb was amputated. Nowadays, we are affronted if we are made to suffer the slightest twinge at the dentist. Similarly an Indian friend of mine asked me recently in amazement, 'Why do you in the West always want to be happy? We just accept.' For her, contentment resided in the ability to absorb suffering appropriately.

A judgement as to what is balanced or unbalanced, healthy or unhealthy, must therefore always be based on an assessment of what is appropriate or inappropriate for that unique person, and be judged from each person's unique vantage point. Our assessment of a patient's state of health will also be relative to what that patient has experienced before, to their ability to withstand pain and to their approach to illness in general. If I have been very depressed and have now recovered sufficiently to function more normally, I might feel that I have regained a measure of balance which to a healthier person might appear still to represent serious ill-health. A person recovering from a bout of migraine will overlook a slight stomach-ache in the relief at the absence of the greater pain, and the pain one person is suffering will be dismissed as insignificant by another. It is therefore not easy to draw up a general definition of what we view as health or ill-health, although in any one culture and at any one time society will set some overall parameters within which each of us can work.

From one point of view, balance, and thus ultimately our state of health and the aim of each life, must be seen as the harmonious flow of the elements within us, and yet I have before me a more charged image, one that is more dissonant, more in keeping with the dynamic movement, the fits and starts, the ups and downs which accompany us on our journey from birth to death. According to this perspective, our unique individuality emerges as the product of tension and abrasiveness; it is the creative result of the differing demands of the elements within us, and, in particular, those of our dominant element.

This seems to chime with what are so obviously our differences, giving our guardian element a cherished status and awarding it great respect. It is here, in this one segment of the circle of the elements, that we are able to express our true nature. The potential within the guardian element becomes the potential for our own growth. Our balance then becomes primarily dependent not only upon this element's state of balance, but also upon the extent to which we fulfil the demands this element places upon us.

Now there are two opposing ways of considering the suffering our patients bring with them, each with implications for the kind of acupuncture we offer. The one is to see in pain and distress something to be eliminated, a hitch in the smooth workings of nature, an imbalance to be brought back into balance. Here a state of disorder is a negative thing. Into this picture we can fit the approach to medicine which sees its main function as the elimination or reduction of pain.

At the other pole we can view suffering as being there for a purpose and therefore as having some function to perform. This emphasizes a positive side, seeing it in some sense as a natural concomitant to human striving. Such a picture appears to make greater sense of our pronounced capacity for imbalance, for it would place it in some context, making of it something necessary. It gives a significance to human troubles. Viewed in this way, suffering can be seen as a catalyst for change, and dissatisfaction the often necessary accompaniment to a human journey through life. For to live satisfied with one's lot may indeed bring with it its own perils, removing the stimulus which goads us towards change. Like the grain which forms the pearl, dissatisfaction may be the spur which leads us on to self-development. For could it not be said that we appear to learn, not from our pleasures, but from our pains?

And yet to these very unhappinesses there is a pattern. They move to their own rhythm, occurring at points in our life where some impetus from outside is required to move us forward.

And they propel us by their prickings towards change. From the perspective of our individual development, they have the potential to move us further along the path of self-discovery. They can lead us towards ourselves, if we choose to grasp the opportunities they offer, for their uncomfortable promptings force us to address often hidden issues we have not yet faced. It could be said that we move in the dark towards ourselves.

And, then, we have to consider how far indeed a state of balance within ourselves is possible or even desirable. Is the aim of any therapy to help a patient reach a state of equilibrium or is it rather to reach their highest potential, which is something quite different? Are the two perhaps incompatible? We can lead a placid, apparently balanced life, and be stuck at some low level of our potential, or we can strive to the highest within us, often fail miserably and yet roam in the more rarefied air of our highest potential, with all the risks this involves. The question here is whether we wish to challenge ourselves or whether we choose to maintain our development within safer limits. The world is full of people afraid to risk change and content to stay as they are, however uncomfortable in the long term this may ultimately be.

Here we see the human capacity for almost limitless expansion of an inner world and its creative impulses as creating the tensions surrounding all those unfulfilled developments which represent our often abortive attempts at trying to satisfy our inner strivings. The constant pressure of these tensions, as the guardian element within us strives to maintain its balance whilst also pushing itself to express its highest potential, makes for an often unsettling life for all of us. Not only do we have to maintain our own inner balance, represented in acupuncture terms by a picture of the five elements circling in harmony within us, but this balance has to be maintained against a background of the strivings of others around us and society in general to express their own needs which may often conflict with ours.

Any therapy, including acupuncture, if it is a valid one, offers the potential for change. The patient is all too rarely aware of the possibly painful repercussions of change upon their life, for changes may be necessary in areas other than those they had envisaged. For example, we may come for treatment to help with a migraine and find ourselves confronting the need to change a relationship or a job which turns out to be the cause of that migraine. Some patients will accept such challenges readily, others will baulk at facing up to what is needed to put them on the path to health. These are often the ones who stop treatment abruptly, preferring to remain where they are rather than dealing with the consequences change will involve.

When we diagnose that an element is out of balance in our patients and decide upon treatment to help bring it more into balance, we are also forced as practitioners to look at what we see the purpose of human life to be. Such are the deep waters of the soul in which the acupuncturist swims. If the guardian element represents the focus and direction of a person's life, then the challenges it presents, and the scope of its potential, must extend throughout that life. The pursuit of the highest each one of us can achieve in a lifetime's efforts should, I believe, be the profound and necessary aim of each life. In acupuncture terms, it is acted out as the development of the patient's guardian element to its highest potential.

And this development is not a one-off thing, beginning at the start of treatment and coming to an end a few months later. It follows a continuous path throughout our life, as we develop and change, and the cycle of the elements turns again and again through each year and on to the next. Each time the cycle reaches the same point a year later it should do so at a higher level, representing another ring of experience added to our life, like the rings indicating a tree's age. And acupuncture treatment, experienced at the highest level, will accompany the patient on this journey through life, sometimes becoming more frequent as stresses occur and more support is needed, at other times infrequent, as the need for help recedes. Indeed, patients willing to accept the challenges of their own continuing development will themselves know whether and when they need support.

Here we enter the complex world of each person's journey of self-discovery. The guardian element is the point in the cycle of the elements where that journey begins and ends. The highest potential each element is capable of represents the range of the potential for a patient's self-development.

We can look outside ourselves for help in dealing with such often troubling challenges, and modern men and women, more reluctant than were our forefathers merely to suffer our fate, often do so, turning to doctors, counsellors, psychotherapists, healers of all kinds, for the help and insights we feel unable to provide for ourselves. We turn, too, increasingly, to acupuncture for such help. And each treatment we receive, if it is the right one, at the right time and given by the right person, can help move us further on our voyage of self-discovery.

Thus each treatment can be regarded as a brief, but potentially powerful, date with destiny.

Assessment of balance

How can the tiny instrument of healing, the acupuncture needle, be brought into relationship with the concepts of individual destiny we have been discussing? And how do we, as acupuncturists, help navigate ourselves and our patients amongst the rocks and shoals which represent the progress of an individual life?

The adjustments in energy which each treatment represents can help a patient's life change course or prevent a patient from drowning beneath sorrows. But the course we help our patients steer cannot run counter to their needs, since one of the comforts to us must be that nature is kind to us, and refuses to accept, except perhaps briefly, interventions which fail to contribute to our patients' well-being. Unlike Western medicine, where patients stolidly suffer often the most appalling procedures in the hope of getting well, acupuncture patients, perhaps because we talk to them in a gentler language of healing, and also perhaps in this country because they usually pay for their own treatments, will quickly stop coming if the well-being they are seeking is not forthcoming.

This is a further reason to be thankful for acupuncture's healing aims, for subtle energies, stimulated by treatment but not addressed correctly, point patients firmly to the door if their needs are not met, providing yet further evidence of nature's beneficence. And, too, we listen carefully to our patients, using their comments on how they feel as one of the ways which guide us to the next treatment. Here patient and practitioner do not confront each other across a professional divide, but work together with the same aim and with the same intention of maintaining the patient's dignity and sense of self-respect. For underlying all treatment is an acknowledgement that only the patient really knows how they feel, and that the practitioner is there to attempt to interpret these feelings, this awareness of what is wrong, into the language of treatment. We all know when we don't feel right. What only the more aware amongst us knows is why we don't feel right and even fewer of us know what needs to be done to make ourselves feel better. This is why we have to turn to others for help, and this is the acupuncturist's task.

We now have to translate this understanding of our patient's needs into the terminology of the practice room and weigh each of these needs on the scales of balance or imbalance. Each assessment we make at each stage of treatment forms one layer in a continuous process of diagnosis, and the corrections we try to bring about with the needle form the individual treatments. Diagnosis and treatment cannot be separated from one another; the diagnosis flows into treatment and the results of treatment feed the next stage of diagnosis.

We have seen that the elements, creators of human life, reflect through the level of their individual and collective balance the state of our health. They also provide the means by which health, once under threat, can be restored and ill-health prevented. The energies flowing from organ to organ, from head to toe, leave imprints of their passing on their journeys through us. They create the flesh and muscle, bone and blood vessel which form our being, and leave impressed upon them signs of that passing. Thus, the jaw can tighten, the head ache, the back hunch or the thigh give way if one or other of the different energies feeding these parts of the body is weakened for some reason and unable to maintain the balance and harmony which healthy functioning requires. Since each tiny fragment of us is a microcosm of the whole, all the elements must play their part in any one action of body or soul. Diagnosing where, in this interconnecting web of actions, one or other is failing to function as it should requires the subtle interpretation of what are mainly sensory sources of information. Signals of distress will be emitted by organs under stress, subtle reminders that attention is required. These messages will travel from the depths of the organs within us out towards the surface of the body. And it is here that we are given our senses to help us detect their presence and gauge the severity of the imbalances they reveal.

We know that each cell forms part of a connected whole, and will thus reveal the balance of the energy flowing within us. This is, after all, how a simple blood test, taken from a drop of blood from our arm, can reveal the presence of liver or cardiac malfunction deep within us. In Western medicine, more detailed analysis of the actual organs themselves, by biopsy of some part of their cell tissue, is required to confirm the presence of such malfunctions. Acupuncturists use equally subtle but quite different means, those of our highly sensitive sense organs, to do something very akin to this. This will reveal itself in what we learn to recognize are slight distortions in the balanced expressions of this element, appearing as imbalances in the sensory signals the organs emit as the energy washing through them picks up their distress.

These are the first warning signs that our energy is suffering, but they are usually overlooked, because they are apparently so minor, and because, too, here in the West, we lack that cohesive picture of body and soul which allows us to connect our sudden bouts of bad temper with our creaking knees, and thus treat both together. For this task we are given the delicate tools of our emotional antennae and of all our senses to decipher the secret messages the elements send from the organs to the surface of the skin. The colouring of our skin, the sounds of our voice and the smells emitted from our pores, all are messages to the practitioner, each message an arrow pointing towards one or other element. To these we add the information from emotional signals we receive. And these messages we must learn to read, for they are the hidden signs of distress which our patients bear with them into the practice room as cries for help.

The sensory and emotional signals are often deeply complex and require time to be deciphered and understood. We are reluctant nowadays to go outside without deodorants to hide our natural smell. We cover ourselves with make-up to hide our natural skin colour and texture. We dye our hair, manipulate our shape in endless ways with plastic surgery, train our voices not to express too many or too deep emotions. All of these are masks we have learnt to put on as the years go by, and have become a convenient way to hide what we feel.

Looked at in this way, very little of us can now be called as natural as the day we were born. So much has undergone some transformation to make it acceptable to the particular society and environment we live in. And, since we must all to a certain extent suppress some part of ourselves in our efforts to fit in with the needs of those around us, the degree of this suppression will reveal itself to an acute observer through some indication of distress in one or other element. We may wish to mask who we really are, but behind our backs our element signals its presence to all who choose to look carefully at us. What we are looking for in our diagnosis is some distortion, an emotion hidden, a colour exaggerated. We rarely see the elements in all their strength and vigour, as they express themselves in a healthy person, and this begs the question of whether any of us can indeed ever be truly balanced. In our diagnosis we are looking for what jars, since the inappropriate stands out strongly, beckoning us to take note. It is easiest to describe this here in terms of the emotional signals we pick up. To the trained acupuncturist, however, the sensory signals the elements emit are equally as important in offering diagnostic information. If I am unhappy but smile, or talk of my loved ones with sadness in my voice, or describe unemotionally events of great trauma, my listener, if he is acute enough, will be aware of something amiss. Event and emotion do not appear to match. Some slippage has occurred, some shift, so that what is below the surface no longer matches what is above. A distortion of some kind has detached the emotion from what it should be an expression of. The greater the detachment, the more this is evidence of some fundamental distortion in the human being.

Our emotions, those sensitive messengers from the depths within us, will have many ways of revealing their imbalances. Each of us will show at different times differing emotional approaches to life which throw a patina of their own over all that we do. These emotional pointers are manifestations of what are seen as the five great emotions attached to the elements which we call by the names of anger, joy, sympathy, grief or fear, each revealing itself as a response, balanced or not, to an element's specific need, Wood's relationship to anger, Fire's to joy, Earth's to sympathy, Metal's to grief and Water's to fear. Since each of us has a particular relationship to one element, we will manifest the particular emotion related to that element as the dominant expression of our emotional orientation to life. Over this we will superimpose other emotional shadings at differing times as our life demands different responses from us. Some of these will be balanced expressions which are appropriate for what is needed. Others will be less so, revealing some imbalance in emotional expression. All, the balanced and unbalanced alike, are diagnostically significant and lead us deep within each patient. Emotions in balance offer appropriate responses to a situation. Anger is appropriate if somebody stamps on my foot, grief if somebody I love dies. Unbalanced expressions of an emotion may be caused by many things. It is inappropriate if a child fails to cry if its mother dies, or fails to laugh when everybody around is happy. These are signs that a child has got its emotional wires crossed, so that its response to what should be joy is sadness and to what should be grief is indifference.

The emotions which a baby feels and expresses so purely, anger where anger is called for, joy where joy is called for, may have had to give way with time, and for many differing reasons, to a gradual inability to express these emotions freely. Perhaps joy unbounded has upset a parent, or anger unchecked has stirred some hidden emotion around the child. Then this joy or this anger have become tinged with an apprehension of risk. The child learns that it may be unwise or even dangerous to allow free rein to one or other emotion. The emotions are being experienced but not expressed and often seek distorted outlets (the smile hiding the hate). Such suppression of our emotion, if allowed no easy outlet, will demand expression in one way or another and has many damaging consequences for our emotional health, leading perhaps to the repressed child who torments animals or the too passive adult. The joy or the anger must be hidden. The expression of emotion no longer matches the emotion felt, and the emotion becomes suppressed and retreats to a hidden area within a person.

We are all familiar with phrases such as repression and transference from our knowledge of psychotherapy. Emotions, no longer safe to be expressed, find hidden ways of coming to the surface. In element terms, the emotions which are the expressions of the balance of the elements within us will reveal their tension and imbalance by the degree to which they have to dissemble to survive. It may have become no longer possible, for whatever reason, for the element to express its true nature in an open way.

An element's subterfuges are many. It learns often surprising ways of disguising its needs if these needs have been trampled upon, developing the ability to transform itself in its battle for survival. Each of us thus proves to be a great actor, taking on a myriad of roles as we try to conceal our true feelings. We can see this in operation from very early on as a little child is told not to hit another when it feels anger, or to give another its favourite toy, when it wants to keep it for itself. Here, these apparently small incidents teach the child that its needs have to be tempered by the needs of those around it, often, it may feel, to its own detriment.

And physical distress has often become the only acceptable way we have to express our unhappinesses. The less the true source of this unhappiness is acknowledged by others, the more it may become suppressed and be released through the safety-valve of our body, a necessary function the body often performs to defuse what threatens to become intolerable deep within us. At the extreme end of the scale is the hypochondriac whose need to express physical suffering, to himself real, however imaginary it appears to others, is so great that in effect it overrides reality. Here, the safety-valve is open all the time.

And thus we may have to learn early on to suppress certain aspects of ourselves. And since the greatest area of our self-fulfilment lies in the true expression of our guardian element's potential, it is here that the effects of such suppression will make themselves most markedly felt. A five element diagnosis thus becomes a form of detective story in which treatment is aimed at peeling away the layers of mask we have laid upon ourselves year upon year. The practice of acupuncture is in this respect close to that of some forms of psychotherapy. We do indeed pay a great deal of attention to the level of the psyche, the soul, for, like the Greek word from which psyche derives, it is the breath of life which animates us, and from which all else springs. Lying at the heart of us, it therefore always has a bearing upon how and why we grow ill, and upon what needs to be done to get us better. These are levels of everybody's experience which touch upon the deepest layers within us, and therefore often expose us where we are most vulnerable.

Vulnerability of this kind is not something we feel safe to show, for we always wish to hide our weaknesses, and thus we learn to don masks. We hide where we are most vulnerable, for our guardian element, revealing us in all our nakedness, has to learn many ways of protecting itself as it guides us through life. Each element does this in a different way, and each person develops their own masking mechanisms. The unique factors which shape our lives and place their particular stresses upon us determine the nature and power of these mechanisms. And the masks we throw up often mask ourselves to ourselves so that we are no longer able to distinguish our true needs and work out ways of satisfying them.

The more a patient trusts their practitioner, the greater will be their wish to lift the masks they lay upon themselves to allow the elements to speak and show their state of balance or imbalance, without fear of judgement or incomprehension. Our responses to our patients will show that we have taken note of the slightest nuances, the smallest hints of unease, the faintest signals of distress they send out. Patients will feel heard and understood, and upon this will be built the foundation of trust which leads us to make a clear diagnosis and enable the treatment we offer to do its work. For the practitioner's soul must speak directly to the patient's if treatment is to address the elements at their deepest levels. Without such a level of trust and understanding, the treatment we offer falls silent where it should speak directly to the patient.

Sensory signals are more difficult to mask at a superficial level than the emotional, and thus often lead us more directly to the element in distress. Different practitioners will find one or other of the diagnostic indicators producing the quickest and most immediate information. For some, a patient's smell talks directly to them, for others their voice or colour. Yet others, requiring time to train their senses, may feel more at ease in the emotional sphere, to which more attention is paid in modern life.

A diagnosis is no static thing. It grows from treatment to treatment. Its tone is set by our first encounter with our patient and reinforced at each subsequent meeting. If we follow the image of the elements here, we can say that a seed is sown when the patient decides to come for treatment. It is fertilized by the warmth of the relationship which gradually develops between us, and out of this there grows the bud of the diagnosis, an initial diagnosis of the element at which treatment will be directed, and a decision about the level of treatment required. Each time the patient returns for the next treatment this bud of a diagnosis will unfurl a little more, revealing the nature of its petals, and confirming or amending the diagnosis. It will only uncurl to its full extent if our treatment feeds the correct element among the five, remaining on the whole stubbornly resistant to the coaxings of treatment directed at the other elements. If we direct our treatment elsewhere it is as though we should be feeding the bud with one kind of fertilizer intended for one kind of soil whilst we are offering it another intended for a quite different soil. It is unlikely to grow further out of balance, but will not flourish as it will do if nourished as it should be.

And now the fruit of such treatment will be visible in the shape of changes and improvements we can perceive in our patients as they return after each treatment. Treatment can thus be seen as the slow unfolding of a flower, petal by petal. It is important to view it organically as something which grows only if nurtured by the warmth of the interaction between patient and practitioner. The diagnosis made and the treatment selected fall on fallow ground if not fertilized in this way. The intimate relationship which develops between healer and person asking to be healed forms an integral part of the success of the treatment offered. When we are in tune with another human being, we become more sensitive to their needs. Our senses at every level are sharpened, honed to a higher pitch. Fine shades of interpretation enable us to see, smell, feel, hear more. And we need such refinement of our senses to do credit to the subtleties of the sensory information each person's organs emit.

Sensory diagnosis

The ability accurately to translate the sensory and emotional signatures the elements place upon us into the language of the elements and then transform this into appropriate treatment for our patients forms the very heart of five element practice. Sensory information evokes an immediacy of response in us, and because of this immediacy becomes a powerful diagnostic tool when our skills are honed appropriately. One of its advantages is that it can bypass some of the complications our minds can strew in our way. There are other indicators to an element in addition to the information which our senses yield, but none of these will offer the reliability of information which our senses can provide once they have been properly trained and exercised. These other sources of information will be of use in helping support our diagnosis in cases where the sensory information has given us an insufficiently firm foundation. For example, people of different elements have a tendency to approach things in different ways, to act in different ways, to make decisions in different ways, even to dress in different ways. The information we glean from such observations is initially less reliable than those provided by our senses, but becomes increasingly significant with experience.

Amongst the physical skills an acupuncturist has to develop are therefore those which involve learning again to use the acute senses with which we are born, but which modern life seems to deaden once we pass a certain age. As infants we detected infinitely subtle sensory stimuli around us, showing by the responses to which a baby's so sensitive antennae alert them that instinctive level of response which enable animals to survive in the wild. But much that is instinctive in animals and young babies has been overridden by the time we grow up. Babies respond to their mother's smell, as do apparently mothers to their baby's, but since no attention is paid to the development or even existence of such sensory skills, they start to atrophy with time. We do not encourage the young to be alert to the changing colours on a person's face, or the changing smells their organs emit. In such a psychologically aware age, we may pay more attention to emotional signals from others, but even here we may be encouraged in childhood to suppress our natural antipathies and distrusts, denying their validity for social reasons.

We lose these natural skills because we do not have occasion to exercise them in our everyday life. If, for example, we are not used to hunting with our nose, because food just sits on the shelves waiting for us, our sense of smell is no longer a life-saving faculty, and soon atrophies. We certainly no longer appear to distinguish our friends from our enemies by their smell, as an animal or baby does, and as one of my near-blind patients still does. Acupuncturists have to re-learn long forgotten skills, exercising them much as a tennis player exercises on the tennis court. We are not trained to observe the changing colours on people's faces or to detect the changing smells on the body, or the changing sounds of the voices as one or other organ shows its unease. Nor are we trained to detect emotional changes, nor even to be sufficiently aware of the emotions that are flying around us, so immersed are we in our own problems. We therefore have to spend time re-learning a baby's instinctive assessment of emotional mood and instinctive response to that mood.

As we build up our repertoire of all these elemental signposts, we will detect the presence of the elements more and more quickly in those we encounter. When we first embark on our studies, the elements are unknown quantities to us, but as their characteristics become more familiar to us, we grow to perceive them more clearly and develop ways of storing all the parcels of information we have gleaned, ready to be retrieved as we make our next diagnosis.

Voices reveal the dominant element very clearly, but again we may not be aware of this. We can all tell from the way a person is speaking whether they are angry or not, happy or not, frightened or not. And we may well be aware of a discrepancy between the words and the manner in which they are expressed. If a person's Metal energy is out of balance, a sharp, cutting note, an edge of grief, may be added to whatever they are saying, where Fire might sound as if they were laughing even when there is nothing to laugh about. Here again, our ears may have become dulled to such subtle distinctions, given the plethora of strident noises with which we are now all surrounded, and thus may fail to interpret the sharp notes or the angry tones correctly.

But a tone of voice which is inappropriate to what is being said, if interpreted correctly, is significant evidence of something wrong. An excessively angry Wood voice, or an excessively joyful Fire one, when there is nothing to be angry or joyful about, are ways in which these two elements tell us that something is not as it should be. They are pointers to distress, just as, in the case of our sense of sight, a certain hue cast over our features points to one or other element, and will indicate the level of that element's balance.

If we are to develop our senses, we have to re-learn to smell all manner of things, look at all manner of things, listen to all manner of things. We try to track down the sensory information pouring into us and learn to categorize it as coming from one element or another, and as indicating whether that element is in a state of balance or not. We learn to look carefully at different colours around us, trying to match a certain tint on face or body to the element which is sending out these signals. We listen hard to voices on the radio, or overheard at the bus-stop, each time trying to trace through them a particular quality which a certain element gives to them.

'Lose your minds and come to your senses', we were always being told by my teacher, J.R. Worsley. There is no truer saying for a five element acupuncturist, nor a more difficult thing to do. The social veneer we all place around us has to some extent to be stripped away to allow us to develop our senses and be in direct contact with our own and others' emotions. This is by no means an easy task for any of us, and our training requires a form of reconnection with the purest, most profound parts of ourselves, a truly wondrous experience for those brave enough to pass through what can be seen as a rite of initiation into our deepest selves.

What, then, are we looking for once we have started to train our senses and look within ourselves in this way? First, we must start to build up a catalogue of references accumulated patient by patient which will act as templates against which to compare the sensory information we receive from each new patient who comes to us. Once we have gained a clear view of the colour white on a patient's face, for example, we will store this memory away under the category Metal in our reference catalogue, and take it out to help us with the next patient whose skin has the same pointers to a similar colour on her.

Similarly, a voice once heard and attributed to one or other element will find its echo in that of another patient, and, by a series of comparisons between the different timbres of voices we have heard at different times, will gradually filter itself down to a particular element. Even if we are unclear to start with as to how to categorize that patient in sensory terms, changes resulting from treatment usually emphasize one or other colour or smell, and this will help our diagnosis. I can still recall the first time I observed a colour change in a patient, just as I remember the delight with which I noticed a change in a patient's mood. And it was through listening to a racing-driver on TV that I first learnt to understand the quality of a Water voice, and through hearing a politician talk that I understood the special timbre of Wood. By such examples, as they have accumulated over the years, I have gradually built up my own library of snapshots of each element to which each new encounter with another patient adds a little.

Of the four principal diagnostic indicators, colour, sound, smell and emotion, some can be more easily masked. Two of them, colour and smell, are least under our voluntary control. We will flush whether we wish it or not, and, however hard we try to smother ourselves with deodorants, we cannot prevent our pores emitting smells. This is, after all, how animals sense that another animal is afraid. Often it is these two indicators, colour and smell, which provide the most direct access to our own senses.

Voice and emotion are slightly more under our voluntary control. Both are ways we have of communicating with one another, and are thus subject from very early on to the necessary manipulations which our lives as social beings dictate. They can to some extent be suppressed, and may only make as true an impact as smell and colour when we allow them free expression. These are rare occasions in the adult, less rare in children whose connections to their emotions and ability to express these emotions directly through their voice have been less stultified by social pressures.

But none of these sensory signals can be totally suppressed even, I suspect, by the most skilled actors for whom control of voice and emotion is their stock in trade. To some extent, whether actors or not, all of us learn to conceal some of the expressions of our emotions, and thus practitioners have to develop extremely subtle antennae which respond to the slightest signal to help us diagnose accurately what is going on in our patients. To the sensitive ear, the sound of anger will resonate clearly even behind a laugh, as will the hidden fear an apparently relaxed person will involuntarily reveal.

Sometimes we are fortunate and come to our acupuncture training with one or other sense already more acute than the others. Each of us will find that we have a preferred sense, some of us smelling things more accurately, others having a better focus upon the emotions patients show. The important thing for acupuncturists is that we acknowledge our weaknesses in any particular area and work hard at correcting them, using our greater skills in one or other area as the main pointer to a diagnosis, and gradually drawing in the other senses to support this diagnosis. In doing this we learn to recognize the specific qualities we know as healthy manifestations of their energy.

There are tones of voices, smells, colours and emotions which we accept as being within the range of what we consider balanced and there are others which we learn to assess on a scale of imbalance ranging from serious imbalance to merely the faintest warning sign of an element's distress.

The healthy colour of Wood is a pale green hue, its healthy voice is clipped, its healthy smell is that of fresh vegetation and its healthy emotional orientation to life is a sense of optimistic forcefulness. As its energy starts to become unbalanced, all these qualities will become exaggerated to a point where they show their imbalance. The green will become an unhealthy sallow colour, the smell will become overpowering, the voice will rise to a shout or drop to an ineffectual whisper, and the emotion will turn into uncontrolled or suppressed anger.

The healthy colour of Fire is a pink flush warming the skin, a sign that the heart is sending healthy blood to the surface of the body. Its healthy voice is a happy one, its healthy smell is that of something warm, like freshly ironed linen, and its healthy emotion that of joy. As it becomes troubled, its skin will drain itself of colour or flush excessively red, its voice may swing from bursts of uncontrollable laughter or become drained of all expression of warmth. Its smell can become that of a hot bonfire and its emotion express too much or too little of the joy which is its emotional domain.

The healthy colour of Earth is a glowing honey colour, its healthy voice has a gentle lilt, like a mother crooning a lullaby, its healthy smell is sweet and comforting, its healthy emotion is sympathy and understanding. When it loses its balance, its skin takes on an unhealthy yellowish-grey tinge, its voice has an exaggerated singing quality and its smell becomes overpoweringly sickly. Its emotion will start to express itself in a range from exaggerated neediness to an absence of empathy for others' needs.

The healthy colour of Metal is a pale whiteish tinge to the skin, its healthy voice is serious, tinged with a grieving tone, its healthy smell is like autumn vegetation trod underfoot. Its healthy emotional expression is an acceptance that all things must pass, to which we give the name of grief. When it starts to falter, its colour becomes ashen-white, its voice expresses deep sadness, its smell becomes that of vegetation left to decompose and it expresses an exaggerated preoccupation with what has gone before.

The healthy colour of Water is a translucent blueish tinge, its healthy voice is like a bubbling brook, its healthy smell is that of fresh water, and its healthy emotion a natural apprehension at the mysteries of life which confront us. Its imbalances place a dark wash upon its skin, its voice becomes choked, its smell reminds us of stagnant water or stale urine, and its emotion turns to deep and often paralyzing fear.

Energies in process of change

It is in developing the skill to detect change that ultimately the secret to a proper assessment of five element treatment lies, for the gauge of its success comes from observing subtle changes to any of the sensory indicators through which we recognize the balance of an element. If we are not offering the elements the treatment they are calling for, they respond with a deafening silence and this absence of any change is as striking and as revealing as when there is change. The elements in effect are telling the practitioner to look elsewhere. When treatment is effective, some degree of change must occur, ranging from a tiny shift to an awesome level of transformation. Such is the complexity of each patient's unique response that we can never predict what will happen, and practitioner and patient await the outcome of each treatment with a similar degree of impatience.

Changes as a result of treatment can make themselves felt in many ways, and a patient's own perception of change also offers crucial information. Here we have to be careful, for patients will react in very differing ways and their reactions will vary at different stages of treatment. In assessing what patients tell us, we must remember that change can be uncomfortable and may therefore be unwelcome to the patient, so that what may be a necessary jolt turning them in the direction of health may be perceived by them as unpleasant. They may have to feel worse before they feel better, but may not be happy to acknowledge this. Similarly, some patients will be sufficiently aware to welcome any change as a sign of improvement, and be unworried by the fact that their backache is still there because they feel so much better in themselves. Others may pin their assessment of treatment on the continuing presence of the stomach pains, choosing to ignore the fact that their sleep is so much better.

Such is human nature, that often, too, patients may not wish symptoms to disappear because this deprives them of the comfort of other people's attention. I had a patient with severe shoulder pains and bad circulation. Each time he sat up on the couch, his lower legs became engorged and turned a deep blueish purple. After one treatment, the circulation in his legs had improved so much that they remained a healthy pink when he sat up. He refused to see this as evidence of any improvement, complained that I had done nothing to help his back and stopped coming for treatment. This is an extreme case of what can happen with any patient, and shows how the practitioner has to have ways of helping a patient deal with the inevitable changes, welcome or difficult, which treatment brings about.

Both patient and practitioner come to treatment with many different expectations. Both may have unrealistic expectations and wish for some miraculous and instantaneous transformation from imbalance to balance, from pain to the absence of pain in one treatment, and will have to deal with the inevitable disappointment when hopes are dashed. For some patients, the concern the practitioner shows them are enough in themselves to make them feel better and return with hope in their heart for further treatments. And this hope alone will help alleviate the weight of their symptoms slightly, which is why patients will often say they feel better just for talking their problems through.

We all have different pain thresholds, too, and different perceptions of what we find unbearable and what we can tolerate. The same headache will not worry us too much on one day, but becomes too intense if we are unhappy at work. Equally, we will each respond to treatment in our differing ways, some impatient for success, others prepared to give their practitioners time. The different expectations with which we come to treatment will make us view any changes that occur from different angles, one person seeing them as amazingly quick, others, like my patient with the bad back and poor circulation, finding them too slow. All these factors have to be taken into account in gauging the degree of change treatment can make, and thus assessing its success.

Tiny shifts in the balance of energy become easier to detect with practice, and may be overlooked to start with. Seeing a change from a muddy yellow to a more golden glow takes experience to detect, as our eyes train themselves to observe ever finer gradations of colour. Equally, the other senses have to be trained, too, and nothing can replace the sustained work required to look at patient after patient in this way. Only when we have seen a greyish-white colour shift to a purer white do we begin to understand what a healthy Metal colour is, or when an exceedingly high-pitched laugh becomes more subdued understand the fear a Water person is trying to mask behind the laughter. In effect, all practitioners have to train themselves to develop the sharp ears of a musician, the sharp eyes of a painter and the sharp nose of a cook.

We develop our senses through observations of our patients and feedback from them. Eventually, we hope we will have honed our senses sufficiently finely to allow us to make very accurate assessments of the state of balance of the elements within our patients. Such assessments, by diagnosing the slightest degree of imbalance in an element, can make acupuncture into a highly effective form of preventive medicine, capable of giving warning at an early stage of problems to come, and offering the means to put these problems right, as far as is humanly possible, by realigning slightly the balance of the elements. Seen from a Western point of view, it is as though we pick up a slight increase in blood pressure and address this immediately without waiting for the hypertension to become entrenched.

And the sensory information may reach us in incomplete form. We may, for example, see the colour red and hear laughter in the voice, see evidence of the anger rather than the joy we might expect to see and gain no impression of smell at all. Here we have two pointers to the Fire element (red and laughter), one possibly to Wood (anger?) and one neutral (no smell). On this basis, we will select Fire as the element we will initially pinpoint because it is the element with the most pointers to it, but we will keep a question mark about the anger, which may or may not point to another element. Is it the forceful anger which Wood expresses, the cutting anger of Metal, the defensive anger of Water or even, as further support for our Fire hypothesis, the anger Fire can show if it feels unfairly treated? At this stage of our diagnosis, we really do not know.

Nor can we be sure that the colour really is red and the sound really laughter, since treatment has not yet reinforced or undermined our diagnosis. This colour and this sound may be masks thrown up by the patient. The most important quality we have to learn to develop is the ability to keep an open mind and with it open senses. We must not lull ourselves into selecting one element, and locking out all the other four. The refinements of our diagnosis as treatment progresses will enable us finally to discard all but one as the guardian element, and even then we must always retain a healthy flexibility and test our diagnosis out again at each successive treatment. Experience has also taught me that my diagnosis of a patient returning for treatment after some gap in time is often more acute because the patient's absence has cleared my mind of some of its weeds, allowing me to see things more clearly and truly.

One of the most rewarding aspects of five element practice is that I am often able to observe the elements in process of change as the needle contacts the point, at the very moment that treatment starts to shift them from a state of imbalance towards a state of improved balance. As this happens, parallel changes occur in the sensory indicators transmitted by the organs through the meridian network to the surface of the skin. As points are needled, the patient's skin may suddenly flush red or go whiter, or a patient may break into a smile or look calmer. These changes can be in any one of the sensory indicators, in a combination of them or in all four.

Changes can be satisfyingly immediate or they may be gradual, so that a patient may notice an improvement in mood only over time. Again, this will depend upon many factors: a patient's initial state of balance (how ill is he or she?), his/ her desire to get better (a crucial and often under-emphasized factor), and ultimately my own competence in diagnosis. Am I seeing things clearly? Is my diagnosis accurate and my selection of treatment appropriate for the patient's needs? In either case, I may observe changes in the elements as I treat, or, equally importantly, I may observe an absence of change, which I will have to take into account when selecting my next treatment. All of these observations will help me build up a picture of the element I am treating, and will help to confirm or amend my diagnosis. No amount of learned information can ever equal what we gain by observations of our own and others' patients as the elements within them are encouraged to move towards a more balanced state through the needle's action.

Observing changes in these sensory indicators teaches us more about the Water or Earth elements, for example, than being told that such and such a colour is blue or yellow, because the change in colour from an unhealthy to a less unhealthy shade occurs within the context of a particular patient, with a particular history at that particular time of their life. The colour will also be drawn together with all those other aspects of the element we have learned about in theory and observed in practice, adding depth and context to our understanding.

One of the difficulties we all have as five element acupuncturists is the impossibility of reaching for a textbook which will help us in our task of distinguishing different colours on the skin, or of defining particular tones of voice or smells. Even when we look at the emotions we all show at different times, how can we describe what the expression of anger or fear is, and how one type of anger or fear may be peculiar to the Wood element and another to the Fire or Water elements?

There is no abstract way of describing green, but you will never forget it once you have seen it become healthier on a patient's skin after treatment. Nor will you forget Fire's emotion once your patient has broken out into a sudden smile as you needle her. For many years I found it difficult to distinguish the yellow colour of an Earth patient from the slightly greenish tinge of Wood or sometimes the greyish white of Metal. I remember to this day the excitement within me when I changed the treatment of my patient from Metal to Earth and for the first time clearly saw a colour change to a yellowish glow and my patient take on that look of repletion, as of hunger satisfied, which I have grown to recognize as the signature of the Earth element after treatment. This was my own achievement after many months of trying to see this particular colour, an exhilarating turning point in my development. Recently, too, I have noticed that I am able to detect more quickly the tinge of fear hidden within a Water person's voice. There have been many such moments for me since then, as there lie many ahead, too, I hope, for this provides the continuing challenge of my practice.

There is one further diagnostic tool specific to acupuncture which I will touch upon here, and which, unlike the sensory and emotional signals, provides a link with a diagnostic technique Western medicine would recognize, and that is the very complex pulse diagnosis acupuncture has developed over the centuries. The pulse along the ulnar artery which Western medicine is trained to palpate for at the wrist is capable of yielding astonishingly accurate information about the energies not just of the heart and its blood flow, but of all the other organs as well.

If we go back to our picture of the energies of the elements circling the body endlessly, we have to add one further concept which chimes remarkably closely with modern chaos theory, where the whole replicates itself in every part, so many microcosms echoing the macrocosm. This offers an explanation for why a single hair provides information about our total genetic make-up, an explanation we can now extend to acupuncture's understanding of the flow of energy circling the body. That flow, though apparently dividing into its separate parts as it creates kidney and heart, bone and flesh, contains within itself all the information Western scientists would call genetic information, enabling these body parts and their counterpart emotional and spiritual parts to form, each cell within us retaining an echo of the whole out of which its divided self has emerged. This echo resonates most strongly where the arterial system emerges from the depths at the wrist, neck or ankle, and provides acupuncture with one of its most specific diagnostic tools, information about the relative strengths and weaknesses of the organs whose messages are carried by the blood to the furthest regions of body and soul. Western medicine in its own way acknowledges this, but in a more primitive form, regarding the pulse at the wrist as offering a specific form of information, at a much more basic level than does acupuncture, where diagnosis of the different energies to be palpated at the wrist forms a highly specific diagnostic tool, yielding much profounder information than anything a Western doctor or nurse has been trained to gather. This highly complex diagnostic tool has very little in common indeed with the more cursory Western pulse-taking techniques.

Each organ sends information in a constant and unending stream through the blood to be interpreted at slightly different sites along the ulnar artery at the wrist, and palpated with different fingers and at different depths. Different schools of acupuncture have developed slight variations in interpretation over the years, but the main components of this diagnostic technique have remained surprisingly constant.

The skill of interpreting the delicate signals sent out by the organs through the blood takes many years to develop to its highest level, but with sufficient practice students after their three years of study have gained enough sensitivity to be able to interpret the most important of these messages and use this information to add to the sensory information the elements show so that they can then formulate a treatment plan. Over the years we develop ever greater sensitivity, enabling us to interpret with increasingly fine understanding the highly delicate signals sent out by the organs in this way. And as these signals change with treatment, our fingers will be able to detect the nature of this change often instantly. We have seen that we use other methods of interpreting change, such as changes in sensory or emotional signals, and to these we add this further diagnostic tool. The accuracy of the information my fingers pick up in this way will guide my selection of a specific treatment, and will then help me assess whether the treatment I have selected has altered the balance of the different energies and in which way it has altered them.

Hard work is required to hone our sensory skills and insights in this way. We can only begin to scratch the surface in the classroom, and after that the answer lies almost entirely in our practice and our further studies. The most challenging moment of all is when we are alone with our patient and have nothing to rely upon but these senses and fingers of ours. How we long, then, for some textbook to reach out for, or some standard treatment to fall back upon. Instead we have to become familiar with that moment of deep uncertainty as we confront the unknown in each new patient. This moment is always there, even after many years of practice, and is, for me, the single most challenging element of my practice.

CHAPTER 3

OPENING THE CIRCLE

So how do patient and practitioner together embark on what is potentially such a profound encounter as that between helper and helped? The relationship we develop with our patients is a very precious and rare one, rare because it is not often that we are granted the opportunity to become as close to another person as we become to our patients. Even with our most beloved partners, relatives and friends, we often feel we must show only a certain angle of our life, else we will hurt or disappoint them. Somebody in a happy second marriage will not reveal much of the remaining pain from the first marriage to their new partner for fear of upset or incomprehension. To different friends we show different faces, often keeping our deepest experiences to ourselves. Only to a person with whom we share none of our everyday existence, with its demands for cracks to be constantly papered over lest our relationships fall into them, can we dare eventually to be truly ourselves. The practitioner, too, is privileged to be allowed to engage in what is potentially such a pure encounter, soul to soul. This encounter starts at the first point of contact and continues throughout the time the patient comes for treatment, deepening gradually as the practitioner grows to understand the patient better and as the patient starts to feel fully confident in the practitioner.

What is initially the aim of the first meeting? It is fairly easy to assume that the patient is coming because they think that acupuncture might help them in some way, although they may not yet have a very clear idea in what way. My aims as practitioner are much more complex. Essentially I have to assess the patient's state of balance, pinpoint where any imbalances lie and decide upon a treatment schedule to redress them. I will call upon all the knowledge I have gained so far to draw together from my time with my patient the outlines of a diagnostic picture within which I will have started to see some of the different shadings the elements colour my patient with, physically and emotionally. The initial encounter forms only the first step in the long and challenging process of getting to know my patient. The treatment itself will be directed mainly at what I will initially diagnose tentatively as my patient's guardian element, and will be confirmed only when I start to see some of the kinds of changes I would expect to see once this element is strengthened.

To illustrate these first crucial few steps I have chosen to describe my first meeting with a patient of mine, James.* I would ask you to follow me into my practice room as I meet him face to face for the first time, bringing with you what you have so far learned about five element acupuncture and keeping this in mind as I invite you to observe me with him. You will know already that I will be seeing him as shaped in body and soul by the five elements which breathe life into him. You will also have some understanding that it will be my task as far as possible to restore balance wherever I detect imbalance. You know, too, that I will depend heavily upon my senses and my emotional responses to my patient to do this, and that what I learn from these will eventually enable me to diagnose which of the five elements endows my patient with his most distinctive individuality, the element I call the guardian element. You will know that it is upon this element that I will focus treatment. You will also have gleaned a little bit about how this particular element can be both blessing and curse, offering its unique qualities to my patient, but turning these qualities into handicaps when balance turns to imbalance.

---

* In all the examples I give, to respect my patients' privacy, I have changed their names, some part of their case histories, some of their complaints and sometimes their sex. None, reading this, would recognize themselves.

Bring all these different facets of your understanding to this first encounter. Peer over my shoulder as I talk to him, listen to him, invite him to share his confidences, build up his trust, observe him closely with all my senses alert, feeling deep within me an echo of what he is experiencing so that I can use my own responses to pinpoint his needs. Observe how James reacts to my questions and my responses to him. Were these reactions surprising or disconcerting in any way? In the story he presented me with, what did not appear to tally, what jarred? Where, in effect, could I see the mask we all put up slipping a little to show the real person behind? For it is here, in the gap between how we feel we should present ourselves to others, and indeed often, too, to ourselves, and who we really are that we will be looking for the patient's guardian element to reveal itself gradually.

And my questioning will touch upon those very areas which we try to keep hidden from one another, or reveal only to those closest to us, our fears and self-doubts, our broken hearts and unhappy childhoods. It takes courage to lay oneself bare in this way to someone we scarcely know, and, however gentle and sensitive the questioning, the initial encounter will put its own special stress upon the elements within us, and in some way force them out into the open by the pressure they are under.

Watch me as I sit down with my notes at the end of the diagnosis and go carefully over each aspect of this first encounter to draw as much information as I can from every detail I have recorded both in writing and in memory. Hear me mulling over my impressions, my perception of what James is like as a person, of who he is, of what he wants from his life, of why he is coming to me for treatment and of what he hopes I can do to help him. Follow my thinking as I assess my sensory impressions, attempting to pinpoint where each element is in or out of balance. Observe the stages I go through as I decide afterwards upon the treatment I will give, and then watch me as I treat and my patient as he receives this treatment.

Participate in my doubts and queries, see how I deal with these uncertainties and then how I translate my thoughts into the action of treatment. Initially the pointers my senses detect may be quite faint, perhaps a hint of a colour or a smell. Each shading taken together with all the other information I slowly gather will gradually provide enough information to hint at one element rather than another. And the picture emerges more clearly once I start to treat, for by focusing strongly upon one element, treatment will reveal that element's importance to the general well-being of all the elements by the way in which it and they respond to the treatment directed at it.

I, too, have to be aware of the pressures upon me. These will include the uncertainties we all experience, patient and practitioner alike, in confronting the unknown represented by each new encounter with another human being. And the patient, as we know, expects much from me. Am I capable of meeting his expectations? What if I fail? What if I prove unequal to the task I set myself, at its highest level that of helping to transform another's life? These, indeed, are some of the demands I place upon myself. And sometimes I may pitch them too highly, often asking the impossible of myself, and thus heading all too easily for a fall and becoming disheartened. I have to learn to temper the demands I place on myself with a realistic understanding of how much it is possible for me to achieve at any one time and with any one patient. The equation formed by patient and practitioner can tilt to either side depending on the extent to which both are prepared to participate in the relationship and how realistic their expectations of each other are. And thus as I greet James for the first time I bring to this encounter much that is uniquely myself just as James is uniquely himself.

So what have I learned about James from this first encounter? James is 45, a father of three beloved children, rather unhappily married for 20 years, but now on fairly neutral terms with his wife. He is coming to me for help with general arthritic complaints in the knees, fingers and lower back. He is very overweight, which has further exacerbated his problems.

He appears to want to test me out, quite sharply challenging me from the start, and I have to be quick-witted enough to work out an appropriate response. This I must have done, and I was aware, almost as soon as I answered his initial riposte, that in some way I had passed a test, for the atmosphere between us settled down very quickly from the rather spiky first exchange to a pleasant tone. Somehow I felt I had manoeuvred myself successfully through some obstacle course he had set me. All of this was a matter of a few minutes, a rapid moment of engagement in which we took stock of one another, he weighing me up as being worthy of his confidences, I aware that he was doing this. In these few moments some relationship had been entered into, a connection made.

What actually happened between us at the start? A question was being asked by both of us, a different one for each of us. He was asking in effect, 'What kind of person are you? And can you help me?' I was asking, 'What kind of person are you? And what help do you want from me?' Each little signal we exchanged, like all the signals between human beings, revealed a little bit about both of us. His challenge at the beginning, 'Goodness, you have changed a lot since I saw you a few years ago', presented me with the need for control. I wondered whether he was hoping to disconcert me and catch me off-guard, for some criticism of my appearance was clearly implied by the sharp note to his voice.

And how was I to answer this, if answer was needed? Here I needed to be quick, decide the best way to counter this criticism by showing that it did not affect me. I could have ignored what he said. I could have laughed it off. I could have shown some irritation. In the event, I said quickly, 'Well, we're none of us getting any younger, are we?', and this neutralized the barbs which were undoubtedly there. He laughed and relaxed, glad, it appeared, to have his challenge met. The first step in this burgeoning relationship had been made in a positive direction. I felt he thought he could trust someone who was not fazed by his directness, as many people must be when they first encounter him. I had stood up to him, and he appeared to like that.

Something of this kind of manoeuvring and questioning is going on when we meet any new person, each of us demanding different things from those we meet. Maybe this patient of mine wanted me to show some flicker of annoyance. In normal social intercourse it is likely that this kind of remark must have proved upsetting or hurting to other people, and if he persisted in this kind of first approach, which I suspect is his manner in general, he will have encountered anger and defensiveness. What he needed, though, I felt, was a boundary drawn by me, and my response was in effect a statement telling him, 'You can go so far but no further.' Once such a boundary was drawn, the atmosphere visibly lightened. He looked more at ease, less prickly, laughed with me and relaxed. His response showed that what I had given him had apparently been what he needed, and his laugh was acknowledgement of this.

To go into so much detail about this apparently small incident may seem a little excessive, and yet nothing is insignificant in our encounters with our patients, above all not those first moments when we engage in the first steps of that initial dance. He had tried to challenge me, testing me out to see how far I was in control of the situation. I had apparently answered to his satisfaction. And from what was mainly a non-verbal interchange I drew much information upon which to start building up a diagnosis.

What signatures have the elements placed upon James, and how does he help illustrate some of the very complex and challenging issues we have touched upon? We will see as we move on to looking at each element in turn that many of the signals James sends out pointed me gradually in the direction of the Wood element. I can see that his skin colour is a greyish green and his tone of voice is clipped and forceful. His smell, initially very strong, showing the depth of his imbalance, is the smell of slightly decaying vegetation but with quite a fresh undertone to it, which is Wood's smell. When he first came for treatment he showed a level of intolerance verging on a general irritability, to which we give the name of anger. He was quick to fly off the handle, quick to judge, as intolerant of others' weaknesses as of his own. He did not appear to suffer fools gladly, as my first interaction with him showed. All of these are indicators pointing to the Wood element.

After a few treatments, he tells me that his body already feels lighter, his fingers no longer turn white when they are cold, the circulation in his legs has improved and his feet remain warm at night. His skin looks healthier, his eyes brighter and he has lost some weight. I feel he is now a little less highly strung and critical, and has become fairer in his judgements. He tries hard not to be a bother, underplays the sadness I feel in him and wants me to get to work quickly to help him, playing down the difficult life he has led and still leads without dwelling too much on it. He does not want to go over the past except in giving me the facts, nor is he worried by the future. Coping with today and ensuring that his family is happy today is what concerns him. What has been is over, gone. He wants to get on with things and wants me to help him do so. His relationship with me is one of mutual respect, but not of dependency. He maintains his right to be my equal but allows me my own area of expertise, clearly accepting that I know what I am doing. He is able to acknowledge improvements freely, of which there have been many even in such a short space of time. There is a simplicity and directness to him with which it is easy for me to engage.

At the last treatment, he climbed the stairs to the practice room with a bounce in his step which both of us remarked upon. All in all, from both our points of view, a satisfactory start to treatment, and one that I would be delighted to see in all my patients. After a few more treatments I suspect he will be off, impatient to get on with his life and glad not to be thinking too much about himself, as treatment forces him to do.

I have emphasized almost to the point of caricature those aspects in his behaviour and speech which later chapters will show point to the Wood element to help the reader see this particular aspect of the five element circle as clearly as possible. To avoid confusion I have not included the many signals sent out by the other elements in James, for like all of us he is composed of all the elements. A touch of red which I saw on his face and the occasional laughing note to his voice initially led me also to question whether he is of the Fire element. It required some confirmation from seeing the effects of treatment to convince me that Wood is his true home. When we move on to the other elements we will see that much of what I have described as significant pointers to the Wood element would not have been there if James' element were Fire, Water or any element other than Wood.

James will always see this world through this particular filter. We can say that, for him, the world forever bears the bright green colours of a spring day which, as we shall learn later, is Wood's preferred resting place.

The elements as filters

We now need to look in a little more detail at how what I offered James in his treatment helped to harness the powerful forces of the elements within him. I have said that the elements create filters through which all permeates to us and through which we and the world outside us interact, and that for each of us one element acts as our personal filter, adding its own colouring to all that we perceive, feel and do. We now need to look at this filtering process more closely to help us understand a little better how the elements do their work within us.

Once again we have to rid ourselves of the Western approach to the human being which regards it predominantly as a thing on its own, as though divorced from the world in which it lives. Physiology and anatomy books, as do the Da Vinci cartoon and the acupuncture chart from Chapter 1, reinforce the impression of a stand-alone body, a cut-out figure which can apparently move to and fro in space as though that space within which it moves impacts in no way upon it or it upon the space outside it.

We know that this is not true. As I have said, if I am transported from England in spring at 10:00 in a few hours to Moscow in winter at 22:00, my body will howl its displeasure, much like some tree uprooted. And to regard each of us as attached like this tree by roots to the ground beneath our feet on which we walk and by many other invisible connecting ropes to the air which surrounds us is an expressive example of the human being embedded in the greater whole that I have described before. Both the Da Vinci cartoon and the acupuncture chart (and by extension all our anatomy and physiology books) should show densely enmeshing lines of communication growing out from our fingers and our toes and from every cell on the surface of the skin towards the cosmos beyond us, through which energy pours towards us from outside, passes through us as it creates us and then leaves us again to rejoin all the energies pulsing around outside us, a vast spider's web of connections enveloping all that exists. And we must not forget all those countless other beings around us, each enveloping us in their own network of radiating energies. We should keep this image in our mind if we are to understand the power and depth of the forces which acupuncture taps each time a needle is inserted into an acupuncture point.

The elements within each one of us, like a personal communication network, are the filters through which these forces focus their attention upon us, and become the means by which their balance is maintained or redressed by acupuncture treatment. Our individual guardian element forms the axis for these forces. It is through their acts of constant transformation that the elements are able to convert all that flows towards us from the outside world into a form which we can use. We use our various functions and structures to change what comes towards us from the world outside into a form suitable for our own use. Physical nutrients such as air, food and water, and more immaterial nutrients, such as the thoughts and feelings of others, alien substances all, have to be transformed into something we can recognize and absorb, and this transformed material is in turn returned to the outside world as exhaled air, waste matter, speech and our own thoughts. Everything, whether moving from within outwards or from without inwards, has to pass through our own personal filter before it can be made our own, and then in turn has to be re-processed to make it available to what lies beyond ourselves.

Our mind, for example, has to process the information we receive into a suitable form for understanding it. I cannot interpret messages spoken to me in Swedish as I can those in English, for I have not learnt the mental techniques necessary to translate the Swedish sounds into those I can give meaning to. Similarly, our soul, so subtle in its interpretation of what comes towards it, has to comprehend the signals others send it in a form that it can understand.

There are numerous mechanisms which we use to absorb and interpret these myriad offerings showered upon us from outside. Everything we take in goes through an intricate process of transformation before it is converted into the life-giving processes which feed our every pore. And each of these pores, too, transmitting its responses to outside pressures, provides information we need to enable us to function and survive. In a similar way we learn to decipher the words that are spoken to us, and to disentangle all the messages our brain sends out to form the words we in turn speak and others hear. All this processed information is directed backwards and forwards from the world outside and inside us, so many signals which our antennae and the antennae of others around us pick up, translate and re-transmit.

In acupuncture terms, all these complex mechanisms are under the control of specific elements, each particular function of the body coming under the sphere of influence of a particular element, and sending and receiving signals from the relevant organs through the medium of specific meridian pathways. Different elements will have differing responsibilities, some engaged in processing our food, others in disentangling the words our ears hear, yet others in responding to emotional signals.

As a simple example of the elements' transformative work, we will follow step by step the processes by which we transform a bite of sandwich into a form which enables it to pass through cell walls to feed our blood in its final manifestation. So let us follow this small and, if viewed aesthetically, somewhat ugly parcel of food on its journey into, through and out of me, and it will tell us a story of awesome beauty. For this is a tale of the creation of life, the life of our cells, from the now dead matter of which this sandwich was made. And this amazing process of transformation continues unceasingly inside our bodies at each moment of our lives. The telling of this tale will also introduce us in greater detail to each of the elements and their specific functions as carried out by the organs over which they have control, as together, and in health so smoothly as to be imperceptible, they weave their differing functions into a unified dance of creation. This will also provide, in greater detail, an overview of the different organs of the body associated with each element.

So here I am holding my sandwich in my hand, and already the elements are starting their work, for my mouth, alerted by my eyes (Wood element, Gall Bladder* and Fire element,

---

* From now on, all the organs of the body as understood in Chinese acupuncture in their widest sense will be written with an initial capital letter to distinguish them from the much narrower, purely physical concepts which Western medicine recognizes as organs.

Heart), is already preparing itself to receive its food. My taste buds (Earth element, Stomach) are preparing themselves to receive the food, and my Water element (Kidney and Bladder) is sending additional saliva and gastric juices to my mouth to enable me to masticate and swallow. All this time I continue to breathe (Metal element, Lung) and with each chewing action I add oxygen and water (Water element, Bladder) to the masticated mixture in my mouth.

My lips and the inside of my mouth (Earth, Stomach) move busily to turn the food over, my teeth (bones, Water, Kidney) bite into the food, and my oesophagus (Earth, Stomach) receives mouthful after mouthful. My Wood element has instructed its Liver to plan when to swallow and its Gall Bladder to contract and relax its tendons to enable the food to be swallowed, whilst my Fire element warms the food to blood temperature.

As this semi-processed food descends the oesophagus and into the stomach (Earth), all the organs involved in its downward journey alert the Stomach and Small Intestine (Earth and Fire) to prepare themselves to receive the food. This is then broken down further as the Small Intestine sifts it into nutrients fine enough to pass through cell walls into the blood on their journey to the heart (Fire) or into waste products excreted as faeces or urine (Metal, Large Intestine and Water, Bladder).

Throughout this journey from outside my body through my mouth, down my oesophagus to the stomach and bowels and back out into the outside world once more, all the organs continue to do their part, planning, decision-making (Wood), warming, feeding with blood (Fire), processing (Earth), aerating, disposing (Metal) and lubricating (Water). Indeed, it is difficult to distinguish between their complex functions, since we are not dealing here, as in Western medicine, with the organs as discrete entities, but regard each as only the centre of a complex distribution network. A similarly intricate inter-weaving of all the functions of the different organs is involved in any emotional processing, but this is less obvious for being less physically visible.

I am describing here the activities of elements all in balance with one another and supporting one another. If any are out of balance, the harmonious flow from bite of food entering the mouth to the nourishment of blood passing through the heart and the elimination of waste products is interrupted. With Metal, this will mean that our breathing may be laboured as we chew, and we may splutter (Lung in trouble), or we may be unable to digest the food on its journey from mouth to stomach (Earth, Stomach and Spleen in trouble), or excrete its waste products from the bowels (Metal, Large Intestine in trouble). Wood's troubles will delay the smooth transition of bite from mouth to oesophagus to stomach and on, as well as interrupt the movement of our eyes as they turn to look at the food, and guide it into our mouth, help our oesophagus in its pulsating movement, and so on. With Water in trouble, there is insufficient or too much lubrication of all these activities, leading to dry mouth or excessive salivation, insufficient gastric acid in the stomach, constipation or diarrhoea. Fire's imbalances will affect the temperature we maintain all these processes at, as well as our ability to sift the nutrients appropriately to ensure only what is pure reaches the heart through the blood, whilst Earth, being our centre, as we shall see, is involved in a pivotal role in all the activities throughout the food's journey from mouth to anus.

We can extend this example to cover any of the actions we take in our life, those of the soul within us as well as of the body. Each requires the harmonious co-ordination of all elements as they help each other remain in balance. In any one action one element may be working the hardest (Metal in taking in and letting go, Earth in processing, Fire in warming, Wood in doing, Water in flowing), but none can function properly without the others' help.

We take the work of these very complex processes for granted in the normal course of events, unless we are dieticians, physiologists or physicians, but they are awesomely intricate, so intricate that I am still amazed at how infrequently, rather than frequently, they break down in us. We can swallow large chunks of food without chewing, eat at unwholesome times of the night, refrain from eating for too long and then overeat, and our bodies usually manage to cope with this abuse, only protesting with stomach-ache, indigestion, flatulence or heartburn when we are unable to absorb the damage to their functions. Emotionally, too, we will initially be sufficiently balanced to offset the risks to ourselves by staying in a damaging relationship or an uncongenial work atmosphere. Eventually, though, the elements will buckle under the weight, and make their distress felt. And we must take notice, for such protests are the first warning sign of imbalance, and, if left unnoticed, eventually of disease.

The messengers of the elements

We now need to return to the site of the needle's action, the body lying there on the treatment couch, and remind ourselves of the pathways of energy running up and down it. As we have already seen, the ancient Chinese gave to each organ a function far exceeding those which Western medicine recognizes, endowing them with personal characteristics. We continue this tradition by calling each organ an official. Each is seen as fulfilling a function in a kingdom, much as officials would have surrounded the emperor in days long gone. Together they form a community, a kingdom of body and soul, in which each has specific responsibilities which contribute to the wellbeing of the whole.

These organs, too, are seen as having developed more complex layers, refined themselves, brought to the fore qualities which the ancient Chinese long ago recognized as spiritual and emotional, making of the Liver, for example, the seat of anger, and the Heart, the seat of love. In fact the Chinese refined this understanding far beyond that hinted at in the West, where we speak of a broken heart, giving each organ its own emotional territory.

Each official is closely associated to the element whose commands it carries out, and represents different facets of that element's characteristics. We have touched on some of these as we looked at individual elements and at the organs involved in the swallowing of a bite of food. It will now be useful to draw them together into a family of functions which act in health to support each other.

There are 12 officials in all, each carrying out one of the functions through which the elements do their work within us. In each case a yin and a yang meridian are paired together, with two paired meridians attributed to the Fire element and one pair to each of the elements Earth, Metal, Water and Wood. There are therefore six yin meridians and six yang. Each meridian relates to a specific official, ten to organs and two others to additional functions which reside within the Fire element, and the 12 meridians thus formed relate to 12 different aspects of the elements' work. The meridians are the messengers which convey the officials' instructions to the remotest regions of this kingdom, and eventually to every cell in the body.

I said earlier that the universe breathes in and out of us in an eternal figure of eight as we inhale and exhale air to feed our lungs. We also inhale and exhale all the other energies which are needed to feed all the officials, making each of us into a very complex recycling plant, not only of physical substances, such as air and food, but of thoughts and feelings, too. The officials provide the different means by which this recycling work is carried out.

We must also bear in mind that the very structure over which the meridians pass, as well as the organs whose name they bear, are created by the energies of the elements flowing through these meridians. What we see as the superficial network of energy shown on the acupuncture chart in Chapter 1 interconnects below the surface with deeper pathways of energy emerging from the organs which give the meridians their names.

It is at the various sites at which the meridian network surfaces on the skin that it becomes accessible to the interventions by the needle we call by the name of acupuncture. These sites are called acupuncture points and are shown as dots along the meridians on acupuncture charts. Each acupuncture point forms an entrance from the superficial network to the structures lying hidden deep within us. They form openings which create tiny foci of energy at intervals along the meridians, and are the places at which energy can be drawn in, along and out of the meridians. Each is a powerful point of access to the energetic network which shapes us, body and soul, each potentially containing so much power that pressure applied to specific points, as we know from martial arts, can kill us, or, as midwives now know, turn a baby in the womb. Each point reflects a different quality of energy, is regarded as having a unique function within the body of points and has been endowed since the earliest days with a unique name which reflects this function.

When viewed on the chart alone, the points may appear to lie at what could be considered random intervals along the meridians. And yet their positioning is far from arbitrary. They are located where the energy feeding that particular part of the body encounters varying structures on its passage around the body, and are sited strategically along the meridian to encourage the smooth flow of that energy through and over these obstacles. Thus there are important points on all meridians as they encounter the obstacles created by the junction of joint to joint and tendon to tendon at important sites such as the knee, shoulder, vertebrae or neck. Points also provide interconnections with other meridians flowing through the same area, so that a particular function of one point drawing energy from one official is enhanced by a different form of energy drawn to it from another official crossing its path at that point. And yet so distinct are the individual functions of the points that one lying half an inch away from another on the same meridian is said to have a completely different action to its neighbour.

Most significantly of all, those areas of our body where we reach out to interact with the cosmos outside us, our hands to the air around us, our feet to the earth beneath us, are covered by the greatest concentration of important points, each finger and toe becoming a receptacle for the energies feeding the world, and in turn through these points creating points of exit to the outside world for the energies within us.

Each tiny acupuncture point will be drawing to it energy brought to that unique site along a specific meridian, and will have a unique action implicit in its unique name. The acupuncturist's skill depends upon translating his/her understanding of these unique actions into a treatment protocol which is meaningful for that particular person on that particular day and at that particular stage of their life.

This should no more surprise us if we remember how one physician or specialist or osteopath will prescribe a particular treatment and his/her colleague quite another. Indeed it is not unusual for one to suggest bed rest, say, where another recommends exercise. To that extent, all therapeutic decisions, whatever their theoretical foundation, are subject to a great degree of subjective interpretation of clinical data, in acupuncture no less and no more than in other disciplines.

Although the acupuncture points have proved themselves over time to be the major sites of interaction between outside and inside, and thus places where this exchange of energy is most focused, each pore is also a tiny interchange site as it breathes in and out. This explains how effective treatment can be carried out to correct imbalances in energy using the many forms of therapy which use manual palpation along the surface of the skin to locate areas of tension, such as massage, whilst acupressure practitioners palpate the same points along the meridian network as acupuncture uses. That is also why we instinctively know that applying finger pressure will help relieve a headache. Our fingers will eventually find their way to an acupuncture point which forms the focus of this pain, and by their pressure endeavour to disperse accumulations of energy there, much as the needle will do in a more focused way.

What is interesting is that the deeper the practitioner's understanding of the potential power of treatment, the more effectively the fingers that hold the needle guide this accumulated knowledge towards the point. We call this the practitioner's intention, and this is one of the reasons why the same point can have two different effects if used by two different practitioners, or the same practitioner at different stages of their practice, the one creating change and transformation, where the other yields very little. The part practitioners' intention plays increases with the development of their understanding of the forces with which they are dealing when a needle contacts a point. The deeper this awareness, the greater the likelihood that the practitioner can address these forces, and tap depths through the treatment which a less aware, less skilled, less open practitioner may deny exist or hesitate to address. At a practical level, the needling itself will be more assured, harnessing energies within the practitioner which draw a greater concentration of energy towards the point. Here patient's and practitioner's energies increase the power of the treatment, the two forces meeting together creating a greater focus than their individual energies can provide. The more aware of the potential within him/herself to influence the treatment in this way the practitioner becomes, the greater this focus.

The energetic system, formed initially of elements, subdivided first into officials, then into individual acupuncture

points, reaches here an awesome level of complexity comparable
to that of Western medicine's multi-layered approach to the
body. If we then interweave into every level of this complex
structure that further layer of the soul within this body, we
build up a symbolic representation of the human being in all
its complexity.

What, then, actually happens when we insert a needle into
an acupuncture point? We start with the understanding that
each insertion influences the flow of energy along the selected
meridian in some way. Amongst its many possible actions is
an ability to boost the flow within the element itself, reduce it,
summon energy from another element to it, summon energy
to address the patient's needs at different levels and summon
matching sources of energy from nature outside at a particular
season or time of day.

The art of acupuncture lies in the practitioner's
understanding of which particular points to select to address the
patient's needs on that day. Different traditions of acupuncture
select the points they use in differing ways unique to them. All
use the needle as their main focus, but to this they may add
the taking of herbs or the heating of a cone of dried mugwort
over a point, a technique known as moxibustion, from the
Japanese for herb. It is as though each branch of acupuncture
uses a slightly different language to interpret what the patient
is saying, although all have a common root, much as both
English and French are based on Latin, and yet an Englishman
cannot without tuition understand a Frenchman. It is therefore
often difficult for different traditions of acupuncture to follow
each others' treatment selections, although all will select their
points from the common root of universally accepted points.

For each treatment I have available potentially all the
acupuncture points on the body, traditionally 365. Many
more points than these are known, and many are rarely used.
In practice, we use only a few of these points, those whose
effectiveness tradition and practice have proved over time. Each

practitioner will build up their own repertoire of points for which they have a particular affinity, but some points form part of the standard repertoire for all practitioners. And each acupuncturist will add his/her own knowledge and experience of the points to the store of accumulated knowledge about these points which has grown up over the millennia.

In addition to points on the guardian element, we can also draw upon other sources. Energy can be summoned from other elements or dispersed to other elements according to the techniques used. The seamless transfer of energy from the Wood element within us through Fire, Earth, Metal and Water and on to Wood again can only take place when we are healthy and balanced, and when all the elements within us nourish us appropriately at the level of body and soul. If this smooth flow is interrupted in any way, one or more elements will show its distress and fail in some way to fulfil its prescribed tasks. The needle can then be used to re-establish the bridge between them. Treatment can also draw on the particular energies in nature outside by drawing to the element some of the energy released at a specific time of day or in a specific season. We mentioned earlier that treatment to offset the effects of jet lag draws on these different energies. Effects will be enhanced if we treat during the season or at a specific time of day or night associated with the element we are focusing our attention upon.

And then there is a large category of those most special points, which have a direct connection to the patient's spirit and which have the power to heal at a deeper level. These points bear names with which they have been endowed since the earliest days, translated in our tradition by words such as Soul Door, Palace of Weariness, Abundant Splendour or Spirit Burial Ground. If selected for the right reasons, they add a different level to the treatment.

In focusing treatment upon the guardian element, we concentrate on drawing upon those aspects of the other elements which will contribute to strengthening this element.

There are many ways in which the elements are unable to feed each other as they should. An official may hold on to too much energy for many different reasons, perhaps because it is itself in need and does not want to deplete itself further, or that it is not strong enough to pass on its energy. Or it may be unable to receive energy from other officials because it is too weak, much like an ill person cannot take in the nourishment a healthy person thrives on. Treatment is then directed at strengthening the officials in question to the point where they can take their proper place again in the overall flow of energy. The point we select for a specific action will activate an opening on to the meridian network at the site of the needle's action. It will have an effect upon the energy flowing within this meridian, within the areas of the body deep within us with which this meridian interconnects and with other pathways of energy as they intersect on the surface and in the depths and interpenetrate each other.

The success of treatment depends, too, upon the existence and strength of that most essential factor, the patient's trust in their practitioner. A warm channel of communication must exist between them through which the practitioner is able to direct the treatment. Both must be in harmony with one another, else whatever effects the treatment is intended to stimulate, instead of flowing strongly towards the patient, will encounter obstacles which impede or even halt this creative flow. If a patient is wary of their practitioner, unsure of them, uneasy in their presence, the body's defence mechanisms will set up a barrier of resistance. Since each manipulation of the needle must be regarded as a form of outside interference in the flow of our energy, however slight this may be and however healing its aim, if we are unsure of what the motive or aim of this interference is, our uncertainty will trigger our protective system into blocking the treatment in some way.

Patients are usually understandably wary of what is going to happen at the start of treatment, and it takes time for the practitioner and the practice to gain a patient's deep trust so that the ground is made fertile enough for treatment to be successful. The speed at which the practitioner is able to translate an understanding of their patient into words and treatment will be a measure of his/her skills. Such an understanding will call upon many insights, and include an ability to translate this diagnostic information into a relationship with our patients which responds to their individual needs.

The practitioner and his/her patient therefore affect the nature and outcome of the treatment given. This is a concept now understood in modern physics where the person doing the experiment is seen to influence the experiment. A needle inserted without regard for the acupuncturist's involvement in his own practice will therefore have a different effect from that inserted by another who experiences within himself at the moment of insertion that connection between himself and his patient revealing both as part of the Dao, the whole.

Patterns of flow

We saw earlier that the Chinese philosophy underlying the practice of acupuncture is based on an understanding of some order and pattern in the universe, and that ill-health can be regarded as some disruption to this pattern. It is pinpointing where this pattern has become dislocated which forms the core of acupuncture practice. We need first to unravel whatever pattern there is before us, make some order out of it, and in so doing make an initial diagnosis of where we believe the imbalance or imbalances lie within the patient before we can select an appropriate treatment. The aim of diagnosis is therefore to detect any disturbance in the order and pattern of a patient's flow of energy. And the pattern we are looking for is centred, in five element acupuncture, on the patient's guardian element and its needs. I have to look at each of the distresses, physical, emotional, spiritual, which my patient reveals to me, and try to place them within a context which reveals to me the pattern of my patient's life. Here, I need to draw upon what I have learnt not only about the nature of the elements and their officials in balance and imbalance, but also about the positioning of the pathways of energy which carry their instructions throughout body and soul, for it is through the energy passing through these pathways that distress will make itself felt.

Sometimes, even for acupuncturists, it is all too easy to forget the deeper, less physical aspects of any imbalance, but they must be borne in mind if we are to fathom the significance of any imbalance, of body or soul, which our patients present us with. Why, for example, does somebody's knee swell or their back ache? A physical explanation will yield some information about oedema or a slight misalignment of the vertebrae. But again we need to ask why the oedema occurred there and then, and whether the displacement of the vertebrae was actually the cause of the pain in the first place. Often the explanation yielded by scans and X-rays may show all sorts of physical disturbances to the body and yet people with very distorted spines may experience absolutely no pain and others with perfectly aligned spines be in acute distress. We would say here that it is the nature of the energy flowing through the spine or knee which dictates whether an imbalance develops, or whether the body remains quite at ease within what may appear, from the outside at least, to be a rather inadequate framework.

I therefore keep before me an image of the flow of the meridians through my patient as I make my diagnosis. I look carefully to see where the pain they are complaining of occurs, and whether there may be underlying reasons which have encouraged that pain to surface there and then on the body. The same is true of any emotional pain. Why then and why this kind of distress? I try to knit all this information together to form a coherent pattern out of which emerges my deepening understanding of my patient's needs. Initially, the pattern is a mere outline, a few notes dotted here and there on a blank sheet. With time, as treatment progresses, the outlines of an emerging pattern which represents my patient more truthfully appear, and when this pattern remains constant, and my patient returns for each treatment in a state of increasing balance, I am ready to hand control back to his/her own energies to maintain. The ultimate aim of treatment is for me to withdraw from the picture, secure in the knowledge that my patients' own energies are now strong enough to offset the pressures upon them, and balanced enough to know when they might need further help.

It will be useful now to look at some examples of how the stresses upon us which we call in Western terms physical illness influence in acupuncture terms the structures we know of as our body and the soul within this body. Perhaps one way to picture this is to follow an incident from its first impact through to the point at which this impact becomes so overbearing that it causes a sufficient level of disturbance to become pathological. The examples given below are aimed at drawing together much that has been discussed before, and provide a practical illustration of how we approach the complaints with which our patients come to us for help.

I will use as my first example that of a patient of mine who suddenly developed severe toothache and asked me for help whilst waiting for a dentist's appointment. The pain radiated upwards to her nose and her sinuses felt inflamed and tender. She noticed that she could ease the pain a little if she pressed the side of the nose. I first tried to place this pain in some context. A tooth may have become sensitive, an abscess might be forming, but why had this occurred when it did and why was pain occurring where it did? From our point of view, any form of pain must originate in some imbalance in energy somewhere within us, and cannot be regarded as an arbitrary occurrence appearing for no reason. I therefore needed to try and unravel some cause for this energetic imbalance.

The main energy pathways flowing over and around the site of pain are the Colon and Stomach belonging to the Metal and

Earth elements respectively, and the area my patient rubbed to help alleviate some of the pain was directly over the last point on the Colon meridian. This point has a direct line of communication with the first point of the Stomach meridian which lies just below the eye. Any disturbance in energy flow between these two officials was therefore likely to cause some accumulation of excess energy around the area in which my patient was experiencing so much pain. When the elements are in balance, energy circulates smoothly from Lung to Colon to Stomach to Spleen and on, but here this cycle had been interrupted.

This filled in one part of the puzzle. The next step was to look at why this imbalance had become sufficiently acute when it did for pain to occur. We need now to look at the particular qualities of the Metal and Earth elements to guide us towards some understanding of why this particular blockage of energy might have occurred. We know that the Metal element is preoccupied with the past, with making sense of what has gone before, and the Earth element with processing thoughts and finding support, a home for us. I knew already that there were pressing incidents in my patient's life which challenged both these elements' ability to maintain balance, and the sudden onset of pain could be interpreted as a bubble bursting to the surface, a kind of release valve, as the pressure grew for her to look inwards and resolve some of these issues.

The treatment I selected helped to bring the hidden conflict within her to the surface both physically and emotionally. By needling the last point of the Colon at the side of the nose and the first point of the Stomach just below the eye, the blocked pathway between Colon and Stomach was re-opened. My patient's eyes flooded with water as the flow of energy between nose and eye was restored, and she could feel the pain drain away almost instantaneously, as though a tap had been opened. Her nose started to feel clearer, and her tooth felt less sensitive to the touch. Within an hour, she could feel no pain at all, and she cancelled her dental appointment.

The relief from physical pain at the needling of these points and the re-establishment of this deep connection between the two elements was also accompanied by a few days of turbulent emotional uncertainty before she was able to deal with some of the disturbance released by the treatment. Significantly, too, she burst into tears a few moments after needling, which both she and I recognized as a welcome release for some of the grief that had been building up in her about her family relationships. Her Earth and Metal elements were now no longer locked in some sort of tension with one another, but resumed the harmonious interaction between elements which we recognize as balance.

The blocking of energy which eventually led to the toothache can be seen as evidence of her inability or reluctance to face up to certain things that were happening in her life, particularly in relation to her home (the Earth element) and what it represented to her of her past (the Metal element). Specifically, the two officials involved here, the Colon for the Metal element and the Stomach for the Earth element, had each been experiencing discomfort, the Colon unable to let go of much unease and the Stomach to process what was going on. The deeper explanation of the toothache provided a far more satisfactory explanation both for me and for my patient, by placing it firmly within a context which represented her at this particular time of her life and on this particular day.

A purely physical approach to the toothache would inevitably have led to some intervention by her dentist of a more radical kind than the delicate needling I had done, and might have failed to alleviate the pain, as we know from all those visits to dentists to whom we go with niggling tooth pain which cannot be tracked down to its source. But acupuncturists in turn have to beware some of the pitfalls which may arise if we take too simplistic a view of illness, and lean too heavily on a psychological or emotional explanation which can lead to some dubious conclusions. This is particularly true of something more serious than toothache, and can produce a line of thought which can lead to statements such as 'excess anger may be one of the causes of cancer', which cast a burden of guilt upon patients already weighed down with dealing with their illness.

The line of causality is not as simple or as clear-cut as this. Would that it were! It is not just one thing, like anger, or an inability to deal with grief, which causes the major breakdown of energies which may lead to a cancerous growth, serious heart trouble or severe depression. There must be a general erosion of balance on many fronts, both physical and emotional, over many years for such a breakdown to occur, and there will always be extraneous factors, such as diet or environmental pollution, which contribute to any gross impairment of the body's capacity to maintain its balance. Nonetheless, as acupuncturists we recognize some initial fundamental cause, buried within the elements, which is the kernel out of which eventually sprouts an ever-increasing level of imbalance and which may eventually lead to a breakdown in the body's normal defence mechanisms. To that extent all imbalances have multiple causes, as the different officials which maintain our health by working harmoniously together gradually lose first some, and then progressively more, of their ability to co-operate.

I chose the example of toothache for its very simplicity, as a starting point for this exploration of how we view the causes of imbalance and their manifestation in body and soul. I take a further example which has a less physical origin, but with its own physical expression. A patient of mine arrived for his treatment in a very angry mood, telling me he didn't feel treatment was helping in any way. His anger surprised me. Up till now he had been a very mild-mannered young man, receptive to all his treatments, and telling me how much they had helped him regain balance. Such a sudden onslaught was so unexpected that all my acupuncturist's antennae bristled. My first thought was 'block on the Wood element!', for as we know anger is the domain of Wood. This patient's guardian element was Fire, and this kind of confrontational anger is sufficiently alien to Fire to put me immediately on my guard and make me look carefully to see whether Wood's energies had become disturbed in some way.

A possible imbalance affecting the Wood element can manifest either as an accumulated deficiency or excess in its energy, depending on whether it is being deprived of energy or is itself depriving another element of energy. The Fire element, through one of its officials, feeds it directly on one side, passing its energy from its end point at the side of the head to the entry point of the Gall Bladder at the side of the eye. In turn, the Wood element's second official, the Liver, feeds Wood's energy directly through to the Lung, passing from its end point at the side of the ribs up to the Lung's first point on the upper chest. A reading of the relevant pulses indicated to me that the flow between Liver and Lung had become impeded, so that there was a build-up of excess energy in the two Wood pulses of Liver and Gall Bladder, and deficiency in the two Metal pulses of Lung and Colon. My patient's untypical burst of anger was an expression of Wood's pent-up emotion. Again, all that was needed was for me to needle the connecting points at the end of the Liver and at the start of the Lung to re-establish a smooth flow of energy between the Wood and Metal elements.

My patient gave a sigh of relief as I did this, a sign that the Lung was now able to breathe in new energy, and he lost some of his brittle, angry feel, becoming softer and less confrontational with me. When we discussed what had been happening in his life in the intervening period since his last treatment, it turned out that he had been forced to confront a situation at work which required him to exercise his authority over a person of whom he was afraid. In effect, his Wood element could be said to have blocked its energies in an attempt to avoid such a confrontation, and expressed its pent-up emotion as anger in a safer place, towards me. In turn, his Metal element, deprived of energy, made him resent the fact that he was appearing inadequate in my eyes by showing his inability to deal with a situation, something very typical of this element, as we shall see later on.

Blocked energies will also reveal themselves through changes in the other sensory signals the elements send out. In this case, his voice had taken on a strident tone, reminiscent of the shouting tones of the Wood element, the colour on his skin was tinged with an overtone of a light green mixed with the white of Metal's imbalance, and his smell was not his usual scorched, as the Wood and Metal elements sent signals of distress to the surface of the body. If we have good sensory antennae, therefore, it is possible for such sensory signals alone to point to the presence of blocked energy. This is, after all, what happens in a way obvious to us all when a person has jaundice. The yellowish-green colour indicates the presence of disturbance in the gall bladder and liver well before the results of medical tests confirm this. And doctors of old, their lack of equipment forcing them to rely on themselves, were much more adept than we have become at picking out such subtle signals of distress, and would base their diagnosis of tuberculosis, for example, on the smell in the patient's bedroom. Now that so few doctors visit patients in their homes this skill has well and truly become lost, but a nurse I know told me that nurses tending very ill patients will know when they are approaching death from the smell. What a pity not more use is made nowadays of such acute diagnostic information.

Each of us tends to have blockages of energy which relate to elements and their officials which have a specific importance to us. In these two examples, I know that I must continue to keep a watchful eye in the future over the officials involved to ensure that the blocks do not recur and to help the patient deal with those areas of his/her life which have led to stresses in these particular officials. I know, for example, that my first patient has troubles at home which will always put pressure on her Earth element. Another patient of mine, for example, who lost a child in autumn, often appears with blocked energy around the Metal element as the date of her child's death approaches, a signal of grief suppressed. To counter this, I have suggested that she make an appointment with me in early September to boost her balance as she approaches this difficult time. The problem, I have found, is that she so wishes to suppress her grief, to the point of denying that it exists, that she forgets to make the appointment, only appearing when her time of stress has already led to the serious bowel disorders which are evidence of her Metal element's inability to cope.

I have used these illustrations of a specific kind of blocked energy where one official denies the next some of its support. These are useful illustrations of how blockages in energy, leading to symptoms of pain and distress, can be dispersed locally at specific sites within the body in this way so that the officials are encouraged to work together in harmony once more. Here, although we may not be treating the patient's guardian element directly, the release of tension in the blocked officials will restore the balanced flow of energy between the officials and thus benefit the whole kingdom of the elements. In so doing it strengthens the guardian element.

If I find none of the kind of blockages of energy I have described above, I will turn my attention to working upon the two officials of the guardian element directly. If its needs are to be met sufficiently to help it maintain a better balance, I have to look at some of the many different ways of strengthening it, as I discussed before. It may be that the energy flowing to the element is not sufficiently strong, and this flow may need to be strengthened, or it may be that it is too weak to carry out the specific tasks allotted to it. In this case, I will need to select specific acupuncture points to encourage a better flow of energy. I may need to encourage a guardian element's mother element, that which precedes it in the cycle of the elements, or even further back its grandmother element, to release more of its energy to its child or grandchild. I can also look carefully to see which particular qualities the guardian element provides which appear to be lacking in my patient, and will select points for a specific patient on a specific day which I think provide those particular qualities which I feel my patient is lacking. The choice of each of these points is a very personal thing, each acupuncturist creatively selecting what he/she thinks is needed now, based upon their knowledge of the patient. Therein lies the mystery in the practice of this art.

WITHIN THE CIRCLE

CHAPTER 4

The Circle of the Elements

And now it is time to turn towards those expressions of cosmic life, the five elements, as they manifest within each human being, and immerse ourselves more deeply in their differing qualities.

There are many ways to approach these five forces of nature. We can write about their manifestations in nature, the seasons, or we can write about them in the abstract, as qualities which encapsulate the dynamics of growth, decay and rebirth. Then, closer in, we can see them through the prism of the human being, with our organs as physical expressions of their actions. And yet deeper within us, we can attempt to describe all those expressions of our inner life, our emotions and thoughts, which owe their existence and health to the creative flow of the elements. All these differing layers provide us with a way into the area of the total landscape occupied by each element. And to these we can add our own growing understanding of these elemental manifestations as practitioners, as patient after patient brings with them each a slightly different focus to our understanding, tilting it a little, adding a little perplexing shadow here, throwing a little more light there.

Perhaps, indeed, it can be said that, so complex is human individuality, we can never truly understand the unique manifestations of the elements' interlinking which define each one of us, even those within ourselves, for are we not often surprised by our own reactions, taken aback by some hidden motive within us, as though missing a step in the dark? As acupuncturists we have, though, to attempt to formulate our own definitions of the working of the elements, however rough and incomplete these may be, if we are to help our patients by using our knowledge of the elements as the tools of our trade. What I write here represents my present understanding of these elements, an understanding modified by each new insight I gain from my practice or from my observation of myself and those around me. I can offer only a sketch, an outline, as a framework within which I attempt to fit patients as a first step in my diagnosis, but it must be taken for granted that each of us in one way or another will break out beyond these artificial confines, pressing our own unique shape upon this basic structure we call the qualities of a particular element, and giving them a distinctive imprint, our own.

And we must never forget that the elements are not static forces, but flow always, changing imperceptibly in a never-ending cycle of growth and decay, and that the outlines we give them can only approximate a tiny facet of this changing landscape of movement, providing definitions which by their fixed nature can never really touch that fluid core of an element's nature. And yet we have to try to enter this complex landscape, however clumsy and artificial some of our attempts at descriptions may be, by sketching the broad outlines of some of the common characteristics which imprint themselves upon those who live their lives within a particular element's territory. It is these which I will attempt to define here in my own way, leaving it to each practitioner and each observer of human nature to fill in these contours further from their own observations.

As I look at each element in turn I bring to it the accumulation of knowledge and feelings and experience which I have built up over the years to form my understanding. And this understanding, like the elements themselves, evolves constantly, as my experience and practice deepen it. If I were to write this book a year hence, much of what I have written here will have changed and developed, however slightly, as I add to it another year's experiences. And my responses are personal to me, born of my own understanding. Others will experience the elements from a different perspective, and each practitioner will use their own insights to form a template by which to diagnose the presence of the elements and their relative strengths and weaknesses in their patients. In this book, I offer my own perspective as a springboard for readers' own developing thoughts.

In our acupuncture practice we see the elements first as they reveal themselves as signs of distress and imbalance, for our patients come to us to help correct some imbalance within them, but we must always keep before us an image of them in the state of balance and harmony we wish our patients to achieve as a result of treatment. And therefore we must first of all gain some understanding of how each element in turn appears as a positive and healthy force of life. The simplest way to do this is to return to nature, where what is within us, often hidden within the complexities of the human being, can be viewed out there in a vivid physical form in the developing shapes of bud and leaf, the ground on which these grow and the air and rain which feed this ground. If we wish to gain an insight into each element's manifestation as a healthy force, we can do no better than to see each as it imprints itself upon nature outside, and, to illustrate this most clearly, upon nature at its kindest, most balanced. For we need to see the general characteristics of each element as being those which have their counterpart in a temperate climate, where spring is recognizably spring, and autumn recognizably autumn, and where there is only one harvest, not two, or indeed none, as in the polar regions or the deserts. Viewed against the backcloth of the climatic changes we appear to be entering upon, as ice caps melt and seas rise, this may seem a little odd, but it is the true, albeit somewhat idealized background against which some of our understanding of the elements within ourselves is built up.

We therefore need to look at what we can consider to be a day in the height of its particular season, Wood's on a bright spring day, Fire's on a hot summer's day, Earth's on a day glowing with harvest colours, Metal's on a crisp autumn day and Water's on a cold wintry day. It is the differences between these varied manifestations of nature which, once deeply understood, will lead us also to an understanding of the manifestations of the work of the elements within human beings in all their diversity. Something of the qualities which nature imparts in this way to what we can regard as an average season forms the most visible entry point into the territory each element occupies within those most mysterious of all its manifestations, each human being.

The ancient Chinese described each element, too, in terms of the points of the compass. They saw them as pointing us throughout our life in one direction, east, west, north, south or to the centre. For Fire, as I turn to the south, I soften a little, bask in the warm glow of the summer sun, start to smile and welcome the world. For Earth and harvest-time, I turn to the centre, draw back into myself, hugging my arms close, keeping what I need for myself. In Metal's autumn, I head to the west and the dying of the year, stepping back, giving myself space, distancing myself from all that is around me. For Water, and the bleak wastes of the north in winter, I hide and melt away, disappearing within myself. Wood, so present in its energies on this clear day here in spring, forces me out into life.

Each element's energies therefore press upon me as the different seasons work upon me, each evoking its own response from me, and each, in its distinctive way, placing me in a different alignment to life and to myself. As I describe each element, however briefly, I can feel my body shift and change in response to my thoughts. Fire makes me feel softer, Earth draws me inwards and with Water I hold my breath. With Metal I move backwards, and now with Wood I move forwards as the future ripe with possibilities beckons. Today, in spring's presence, I can feel the pull of Wood's energy as it turns me towards the east and the rising sun, awakening in me something of the excitement and vigour all that is new brings with it. With this element I look forward into the future as though readying myself for action.

There is a force which shapes us, drawing us out of the undifferentiated mass of the non-living into a form all our own, an outline within which we act out each our own individual life. To this energy the ancient Chinese gave the name of the element Wood, that which propels us into our existence and provides the boundaries to prevent that force from dissipating itself. With Wood, then, we start our exploration of the shaping of a human being, moving out on to a landscape of hope and the future before us.

CHAPTER 5

THE WOOD ELEMENT

It is spring now. Out of the deep darkness of winter light is breaking through. Nature is starting to expand, breathe out, with each breath expelling from each of its pores manifold buds, like tiny hibernating animals emerging from their burrow. They are so tightly coiled, those dark twigs, dead, lifeless, which held to themselves their winter secrets, now coaxed slowly by the growing warmth of the sun to emerge first as slight bumps and indentations along the smooth boughs, then as cuts breaking the surface to allow glimpses of brightness, then finally the whole bud, a small explosion, a signal of life renewed, death conquered, the future made possible, safe in its new hands.

The excitement of it! The buzz and hum of expectation as though those myriad stirrings beneath the soil and in the bough send out messages, forerunners announcing multitudinous moments of birth throughout the world. And then the shimmer of green, always green, that first unleashing of this colour of hope against the dark branches of winter. A delicate coating, placing round twig and branch a breathless haze of colour, at first only a pale adornment, a slight touch of life, then a greater flowering as the buds take on each their own individual colouring, breaking open to release glimpses of white, blue, red, yellow, before finally revealing myriad permutations of colour, each shading offering a glimpse of new life.

Today amongst a bank of rhododendrons one is starting to show its true colouring. The others remain mute, not yet warmed sufficiently by the sun. By tomorrow, I expect, another and yet another will burst their buds open. There is still a chill in the air, warning the buds not to fling open their arms too rashly before the sun starts to warm the land as the days lengthen. The world expands, with relief throwing off its winter chill.

There is no better time, I feel, to start this exploration of the elements, as I wander underneath bud-laden trees on a bright spring day. Life around me is buoyant, children chasing balls, dogs jumping, runners running. The very air seems alive with such vibrancy that I, too, respond by a quickening of the pulse and an impatience in my stride as though there is much that I have to do. And yet I don't know quite what it is and where to start. And, until I started writing this, even with which element to start. But the strong pressure upon me of all this emerging energy out here has its own imperative and I cannot deny this, and thus, with Wood, the element bearing down upon me today, I have started.

Spring always disturbs me, makes me dissatisfied and fractious as though I am being pushed along against my will I know not where. It will take a few more spring days like this to settle me down and give me direction. I am rattled out of the old of winter, its familiar darkness and shortness of day, into the new of spring and I feel within me that shock of the new. There is power here strong enough to push me unwillingly forward out of winter's stagnation. For other people, though, and I expect for many of those reading this book, spring has quite a different impulse behind it, proving a welcome advance rescuing them from the inertia of winter. For these, the force of spring wafts them eagerly forward.

Here we see two differing perceptions of the same force, the one finding it disturbing, the other welcome. Each of us will have similarly differing perceptions and reactions to the actions of the individual elements. And those who find the advent of spring somewhat threatening, as I do, will be threatened by its energy each in a different way, just as those who breathe a sigh of relief as the days lengthen will each be relieved for a slightly different reason. For each of us a particular source of energy may be a more or less creative force, another a more or less negative force. What each phase of energy brings to us will affect each of us differently, and these differences, too, will vary depending on the overall balance of the different energies within us at that particular point in time and will also have their own daily and seasonal variations.

To some extent each element is subject to its own laws and speaks its own language. For a person with Wood as their element to speak to a Fire person is indeed for each to speak a slightly different language with its own inflections, its own vocabulary and its own particular emphases. For a brief time during the season which relates to each particular element, as that element's energy flows more strongly within us, we all speak something approaching the same language. Thus today, out here in the spring sun, I am more at one with those who have Wood as their guardian element than at any other time in the year. For these few weeks we will speak something approaching a common language, imbued with the thrust and power of spring. Briskness and vigour in all that we do are the order of the day.

If we were to listen very carefully, too, we would also hear in all our voices the slightest echo of that shouting note we characterize as Wood's tone, a slightly more emphatic note, as we absorb some of Wood's strong energy into our speech. It is as though the renewed power in nature unleashes within us just a tiny spurt of more forceful energy. Wood people will feel these effects most strongly and respond to their own element's seasonal stimulation more negatively or positively depending on their state of balance.

What do my own feelings of disturbance have to tell me about the Wood element? I can feel that something deep inside me is responding to some stimulus. My emotions are stirred and I have become slightly uneasy and unsettled. If I translate this into the language of the elements, I now see that the phase of energy in nature we call spring, the product of the

Wood element in nature, has stirred awake some corresponding response within me, both physically, in that I find myself moving more briskly and looking around myself more eagerly, and emotionally, in that that deepest part of me is disturbed. Both body and soul react to some outside stimulus.

Something of Wood's force is stirring in me today, challenging me forward on some path I need to follow, making me impatient. My Wood energy is demanding something of me, forcing me in some new, as yet unclearly defined direction. Some new bud within me is starting to open. There is a part of us, too, which is always thus budding with hope. It is the starting point of all things, the new-born, the hopeful, the east, the rising sun, the bud on the tree, the spring of the year and the spring in our step. We all have this energy, and it flows through its own pathways within us, instilling in us hope, making us energetic and forceful, drawing us out from the passivity of winter into a new world where hope springs eternal.

Picture the immense flatness of a winter landscape, snow-covered, dead, frozen, no glimmer of life to relieve its pall of death. How indeed could life have survived below that cold girdle, clasping all things tight to the earth in its stranglehold? And yet, deep in the bowels of that inert landscape, a force, which we call by the name of Wood, endlessly budding into hope and renewal, stirs into life. And that is indeed the miracle of it, because that little bud fighting its way through the hard crust of winter is our only sign that the seed of life has remained alive awaiting the moment to renew itself. Little wonder, then, that Wood is forever hopeful, the eternal optimist, with a belief that all things are possible. For indeed, if it can coax life from the death of winter, to Wood nothing can seem impossible.

Its vigour and power set no limits to what it feels it can achieve, for wherever it looks there are jobs to be done. Many might well baulk at the tasks Wood sets itself. If everything is possible, how much, how infinitely much, there is, in its eyes, to do. And that is why it is so terribly busy. How could it possibly stand still whilst there is so much out there still remaining undone? It is its task to be there at every start, for without it nothing could grow. Unceasingly it shoulders its burden and starts off again, for all things await its life-giving thrust. Wood brings into being all that which might otherwise have remained part of the undifferentiated mass of the non-living. It provides shape for the shapeless, and gives form to what is yet unformed.

The emergence of just one tiny bud, out of the millions upon this earth, as it tears its way out of the lifeless sheath of its twig, reminds us of the focused strength required for the renewal of life. The force inside that bud propelling it forward into life is strong enough to break through the dead and frozen earth. Life wants to be lived, and very little can stay its progress, and yet Wood must set the limits of what is possible upon what is potentially unlimited, as it concentrates all its force upon each single act of creation.

Forcefulness, singleness of purpose and control are required somehow to concentrate enough energy at that one spot of all the possible spots in the universe for life to restart in the shape of a single bud. And strength and vigour are the true domain of Wood, inertia and entropy its enemies. It is forever battling, for it represents our spring-time, and spring is in eternal combat against the dark forces of winter, which try to pull us down, deep down, into perpetual sleep.

A bud thus bursting its way out imitates the convulsions of childbirth. Wood is, and has to be, a violent element. It has to tear us from the comfort of the past into the future, from the familiarity of what we know into the unfamiliarity of the unknown. In so doing it ensures our survival, for without its energy we would remain a dead planet. And just as a tree retains for its lifespan the imprint of that first bud from which all its future growth has come, so Wood's buds remain deep within us, as we emerge above ground from the winter of non-existence, each a tiny shoot bearing within us the imprint of all that we will become.

Wood is above all a doer, a setter-in-motion, getting things under way. The clenched fist, so typical of this source of energy, symbol of the clenched energy tightly sheathed within a bud, signifies the desire and the power to do things, and can translate itself into the clenched fist of anger if these things do not get done. There is a push behind all that Wood does, a concentrated focus aimed at one thing only at a time, the doing of which is its function. Its potential is for constant expansion, constant activity, the shaping of things for its own end.

Each element is showered with blessings and curses. Wood's blessings are its tireless capacity for activity, an insatiable curiosity and a need to get its own way, allied to, and sometimes overridden by, a reluctance to allow others to do what they want, a restlessness of purpose, and a lack of focus where focus is most needed. Its energy can become unbridled, its expansive drive hemmed in or so uncontrolled that creative action dissipates itself into a kind of aimless frenzy. We see this overprofusion in spring outside when gardeners have to cut back excessive growth to contain the plant and enable it to flourish within appropriate boundaries. The force to get things going and then to rein them back sufficiently is the quality of energy Wood offers the other elements. When present in all its power, Fire, Earth, Metal and Water depend upon this ability to initiate and then control the explosion of all things as they start. This is the kernel of Wood's contribution to the cycle of life.

But if the plans for its own growth are blocked, the forceful optimism which is its hallmark will change into the frustrations of impeded growth. Imagine a bud forbidden to open, remaining forever tightly folded in upon itself. Thus Wood out of balance. And this is where imbalance and illness creep in, for if a sudden frost can destroy the buds on the trees, so, too, can the chilly winds of life shrivel the buds within us, preventing our unfolding. The endless struggle between the forces of inertia which attempt to lure us with their soft murmurings towards laziness and inactivity, and the forces of life goading us to work, takes place on a different battleground for each element. Each can turn the fertility of its gifts into sterile growth. Wood can turn upon itself, nipping itself in the bud.

And thus Wood, the great giver of hope, can itself start to lose hope, the energy and vigour with which it sets to work seeping from it. This strong element weakens at its own roots, and as its strength ebbs from it, it loses direction. The sense of aimlessness, always potentially there within it as its dark side, is the burden it has to carry, for if it is not strong enough, it loses its capacity to move us towards the future. Hope can turn to hopelessness. And then it will work only sporadically, its bursts of vigorous activity interspersed with discouraging periods where it can do nothing. Its strong limbs accustomed to striding purposefully towards the future, become muscle-bound, unable to move, where movement is so greatly required of them. Rigidity takes the place of flexibility.

Wood's buds remain there deep within all that we do, just as a tree retains for its lifespan the imprint of that first bud from which all its growth has come. Within every action we take is the bud which first sets it in motion. Within every thought that we think is the bud which first reveals that thought to us. Within every feeling that we have is the bud which first starts us having that feeling. The eternal starting point of all things is that to which the Chinese have given the symbol of the element Wood.

The signatures of Wood

We now need to extend our understanding of the Wood element a little more by looking at the signatures it places upon us. I have said that this starting, budding part of us, like the true gardener that it is, lays a green finger upon us, imprinting upon our faces the pale green hues of the springtime. We can also smell the imprint of this element which gives our bodies the fresh smell of the morning dew upon leaves, a lightness very unlike the heavier smells of nature in summer (Fire) or late summer (Earth). Our voice, too, will bear its imprint as it tries to stamp its authority on whatever it says, its sharp and staccato sounds so many attempts to control the world and bend what it can see as chaos to its desire for order.

We have to learn to recognize each of these sensory signatures by training our ears, eyes and nose to perceive their different manifestations. Words alone can do nothing to help this learning process, for they cannot convey the subtleties of a distinctive smell, the strange emphasis to a voice or the fluctuating colours upon a person's face. I can offer a few examples of some of these signatures upon famous people, but until we have the evidence of our own senses we cannot develop the necessary sensitivities of perception. With emotional signatures, however, we enter a different territory where we touch upon areas deep within each of us for which the written word has the ability to evoke resonances common to us all. I can write here, as I will do, about Wood's emotion, anger, in ways which will, I hope, have meaning for those who read this in a way no description of mine of colour, smell or sound can do.

It could be said that the word emotion, traditionally associated with an element, is almost too narrow truly to reflect the extent of an element's influence upon an area of activity involving that deepest part of us, our soul. Here, with the emotion associated with the element Wood, we touch upon our being's efforts continually to express our own individuality in a world teeming with many millions of others of us trying to do the same, each of us a tiny bud determined to force our way out towards the light. And the strength which buds are able to call upon in their efforts to break apart the thickest concrete or stoniest ground on their climb towards the sun is reflected within us in the strength we can summon from the Wood element both within and outside us as we attempt to assert our right to be uniquely ourselves.

The emotional sphere within which Wood operates is that which we describe, inadequately, as all descriptions of emotions must be, by the word anger. It is that part of the emotional spectrum where those with Wood as their guardian element are most at ease and if, challenged, where they will take refuge. It is Wood's familiar emotional resting place. It is only an adequate description if we use the word anger in its widest sense, without the negative overtone often associated with the word. In its widest, most creative sense, it is a form of necessary emotional forcefulness which we must all be able to call upon if we are to assert our right to be ourselves. When balanced, we express this emotion naturally by not allowing others to stand in our way physically or emotionally. It enables us to stand up to them if they try to block us or push us aside. We act forcefully where force is needed, and we control ourselves where force is not needed. Balanced anger is the power we find within ourselves to prevent others denying us the right to do what we believe we need to do. It is the emotion aroused in us as we confront vigorously what is impeding us. Such confrontation is necessary if we are to survive, for it is only in this way that we can force aside those who try to halt our progress.

Anger can also be a negative expression when its response is out of proportion to what is required. If somebody stands in your way on the street so that you cannot pass, you have a right to ask them to move aside and to express anger if they do not. If you shoot them instead, your anger is out of proportion to what is appropriate. It is also shortsighted, since you may well find yourself marched off to prison where your desire to get your own way will now be totally circumscribed, a compelling example of how our imbalances lead to results which are the very opposite of what we intend.

We all know what it is like to be angered by such frustrations. We are then like buds forbidden to unfold, and if we are thus denied for long enough, the colour of our life may take on a constant tinge of anger, as though the inhibition to our growth has become a permanent burden to which this anger has become our only reply. We will each have our own way of expressing anger, and this will depend on the state of balance or imbalance of the Wood element within us, and thus the advent of spring, evoking its strong echo within us, will affect us all differently, depending upon our emotional state of health. It will uniquely reflect this element's balance within us. Some of us may be stimulated by the need to combat another's anger vigorously, others defeated and cowed by it. Some will hide their own feelings of anger rather than expressing them openly, whilst yet others will allow free rein to their irritation. And at different times and in different circumstances our responses will be less or more extreme.

We can describe those experiencing their anger freely but appropriately where anger is needed as allowing their Wood element to expand, those denying this anger expression as inhibiting their Wood element. In assessing how balanced a person's relationship to the Wood element is we have to judge whether the overt expression of anger or its denial are appropriate responses at that particular moment in that particular situation. And then we need to look at Wood's dominant position in those who have it as their guardian element. Here, the whole direction of their life, if it is lived productively, can be said to find its fulfilment in that one segment of the cycle of the elements, and they thus have a particular relationship to the energies in nature which flow in springtime, and to the forcefulness these energies evoke.

Anger can also be suppressed, and this is just as much evidence of imbalance as its overt expression can be. We may choose hidden ways of asserting ourselves, because life has taught us that it is unsafe or unwise to express our own wishes so openly. And thus we may learn to drive our anger underground, because society frowns on adults who express their wishes too stridently, forcing us to suppress what should be expressed openly. If anger is suppressed for too long, this may turn us into those who enjoy seeing others break rules we ourselves dare not break, often secretly encouraging them to do so. This allows us to bask in the reflected glow of the anger these others will evoke, whilst standing outside the range of any possible repercussions.

The suppression of our right to express our needs openly may be the motivating force behind a person's desire to work in an environment where such suppression is built into the system, such as in a rigidly authoritarian community. For if deprived of the power to order the universe as it wishes, Wood has to look to others for that very order and structure it should itself provide. It may also be one of the reasons we all enjoy thrillers so much, experiencing vicariously, from the safety of the armchair or the cinema seat, the antisocial behaviour and the uninhibited acting out of others' anger, through the crimes committed by the baddies, and at the end of the book or film reassuringly returned, through the actions of the goodies, to what society considers acceptable.

What we see here are examples ranging from one side of the spectrum of self-assertion to the other, from the balanced expression of a person's right to be allowed to unfold according to their inner imperative, to the disturbed expression of this same need, becoming finally a denial of self, and an infringement of the rights of those around. We see this clearly in the actions of someone the worse the wear for drink who ends up denying both himself and others the right to enjoy themselves by engaging in a fight or falling over drunk. Here alcohol may be seen as stifling the Wood element's ability to stay in control and know where it is going, whilst at the same time that need to stay in control becomes so extreme that the drunk person dominates the company he is in, holding everybody in thrall to his antics, whilst allowing himself absolute freedom, untrammelled by any social qualms, to do what he wants, say what he wants and act out his anger exactly as he chooses.

Here is an example of Wood's energy gone wild, crushing all around with its power. Focus has been so totally suppressed as to make it impossible for the alcoholic to stand up, let alone control his limbs or speech or move in any direction at all, physically or spiritually, a sign of Wood's inability to control its ligaments and tendons. The bud is indeed withered on the bough, but as it withers it tries to deny others the right to unfold as they wish.

Interestingly, too, by acting in this way, the drunk person succeeds in creating the emotional atmosphere in which the Wood element feels most at home, for nobody in the presence of such behaviour can fail to feel stirrings of anger at having their right to proceed in life circumscribed by such antisocial behaviour. The shouting, fighting and general interruption of the activities of others which this involves stokes up in others the very emotion with which the Wood element is most at home, that of anger.

Alcohol, as we know all too well from Western medicine, also harms the liver, and here for a time Chinese and Western medicine walk side by side. We have seen that each element creates different organs of the body. The two Wood officials are the Liver and Gall Bladder, both actively involved in detoxifying alcohol. Over-consumption, by harming the liver, will throw the Wood element further and further out of balance, and as it does so it sends out messages of ever increasing distress.

In states of imbalance, all Wood's sensory indicators will become increasingly exaggerated so that the extreme alcoholic will swing rapidly from one state of anger to another, just as the skin colour will become a sickly greenish-yellow shot through with the red of the Fire element. This we will see later is connected to Wood as child is to mother. What Western medicine diagnoses as cirrhosis of the liver, Chinese medicine sees as an extreme level of imbalance in the Wood element, as expressed in its organs, the Liver and Gall Bladder.

We can see now a little more clearly how that sense of constant movement and expansion which is visible as spring bursts into life is mirrored within each of us by the effervescent bubbling of all the activities which enable even the tiniest movement of body or soul to take place. And yet all this seething activity is contained within the few square feet of our bodies, each of these movements circumscribed by the space allowed it to expand and then to contract. Where it is not thus circumscribed, as we have seen in the case of the drunkard shouting and hitting out, we can see the force behind all Wood's actions unleashed now on to the world outside in an uncontrolled explosion, the fist knocking us over, the verbal abuse experienced, too, as a physical blow.

Wood's two officials

It will be useful now to look at the action of Wood's two officials, the Liver and the Gall Bladder, as they do their work within the human body and soul. We can approach this by looking in detail at an example of their actions as they carry out what might appear the simplest of tasks, that of helping us make a cup of tea. And this illustrates, perhaps in a surprising way, how complex are the intricate activities involved in such apparently simple actions.

First, it is important to give these two officials the titles by which they have been known since the earliest times, and these indicate their functions. According to the ancient Chinese, the Liver is the official in charge of planning in the kingdom of body and soul, the general on the field of action, and the Gall Bladder, the official in charge of decision-making, the field commander carrying out the general's actions. The Liver is yin, inward-dwelling, the general in his tent, the Gall Bladder, yang, outward-looking, ready to spring into action at the Liver's command. At a physical level they both control the actions of our ligaments and tendons, so that our movements are co-ordinated.

A few moments ago I was sitting writing this and found my thoughts slowing down. 'Time for a cup of tea', I said to myself, got up, made myself one and settled down again at my desk to write these last paragraphs. If I analyze what happened in those few minutes, I find that there are many complex actions involved in what appears to be such a simple action.

I had to lay down my pen, push aside my chair, straighten my back, push myself to my feet, get these same feet and then my knees and hips and upper body together to make a concerted effort to engage in the complicated movements we call standing up and walking, plan to stop myself when I reached the sink so as not to knock into it, fill the kettle up to the required level but not overfill it, turn it on, move to the cupboard to take out a cup, move to the fridge to take out the milk, move to the store cupboard to take out the tea, open the box of tea bags, select one, return to the kettle for some boiling water, remove the teapot lid, pour a little but not too much boiling water into the teapot to warm it, swill it around, pour it out, move back to the kettle, put it back on so that it reaches boiling point again, place the teabag in the teapot, fill the teapot with water, replace the teapot lid, wait a few minutes, stir the teapot again, fill up a cup, remove the cap from the milk bottle, pour a little but not too much milk into the cup, replace the cap, open the fridge door, replace the milk in the fridge, close the fridge, go to the drawer, remove a teaspoon, place the teaspoon on the saucer, take the cup and saucer in my hand, turn towards the desk, guide my feet, knees, hips and upper body to move towards the desk, bend them to place the cup on the desk, then bend them in a different way so that I can sit down on the chair, put my hands on the sides of the chair to draw it nearer to the desk, and then at last reach out for the cup and take my first sip.

In all these actions, commands are speeding from limb to eye, to mind, to brain and back to initiate and complete a dizzying display of co-ordinated activity. The mere writing down of all these actions now exhausts me, and yet when I carried them out I did all that I have described without the slightest conscious awareness of all this activity going on inside me and without any sense of tiredness. And this description only sketches what my body had to do to complete this one simple but intricate performance. I was not at the same time, as an actor would be on the stage, delivering a powerful performance as I move around, where in addition to the physical actions I was taking I would also have had to draw on Wood's help to articulate my words and the emotions they contained.

We are usually unaware of what is involved in moving ourselves around, as I was doing then, unless we are a little baby learning these movements for the first time, when we need months of concentrated effort before we are able to bring all these differing actions under sufficient control to focus first our eyes, then our hands, then every limb to enable us to grasp, sit, crawl, stand, walk and finally run. And it takes even longer for a child to learn to talk and express its thoughts coherently. For those who lose the use of functions which affect co-ordination, perhaps as a result of a stroke or a car accident, the efforts required to re-learn how to co-ordinate all these multiple activities are immense, as their Wood element tries to set in motion again all this concerted activity to which it has lost the key. In acupuncture terms we would say that it has to re-educate the Liver and Gall Bladder, among many other officials involved, in the planning and decision-making involved in moving their limbs.

The Wood officials lie at the heart of all this buzz of activity, deciding first that I wanted this cup of tea and then which action I needed to select to enable my toes to balance themselves so that I remain upright, my eyes to judge the distances in front of me so that I place my cup gently on its saucer and not with a crash, my fingers to grasp the cup to lift it to my mouth, the time at which I decide the tea is too cold now to drink. Each of these actions requires orders to be sent to my tendons and ligaments to tighten and relax, tighten and relax, and to my brain to tell me what I need to do next. If we were to freeze-frame me as I move from my desk to get my cup of tea and back again, we would see each part of my body doing a great number of intricate movements and adjustments before I sit back in my chair. And within myself these movements are replicated by the many instructions I am sending forth as I monitor my frustration at finding my thoughts drying up. Here the same ferment of activity which the getting of my cup of tea set in motion is continuing inside me, as I turn my thoughts around in my mind so that I can view things from a different angle.

All these activities of body and soul jostle together in a constant dance of movement co-ordinated by my Wood element as it directs the tiniest cells within me to coalesce together so that my tendons and muscles can draw my back up straight or relax a little, my mouth sip my tea or my thoughts flow from deep within me on to the page. This vast array of potential movements under Wood's control awaits the commands of the Liver to plan ahead what needs to be done and the commands of the Gall Bladder to set about doing these things.

This describes only one small activity spanning maybe 15 minutes, a mere one hundredth of all the quarters of an hour we spend on the many different activities which cover one day. It must be remembered, too, that all the other officials are active at the same time, and here we are only describing what two out of the twelve do. It amazes me that the intricate interweaving of all these myriad acts carries on imperceptibly, in health, and only becomes perceptible when, as we are doing here, we break them down into some of their component parts, or when it itself breaks down through some imbalance in one or other official.

We saw some small example of this in my description of the journey of a bite of food into, through and out of us. If we expand this to cover all that we do at any hour of the day, every day of the year and every year of our life, this opens us on to a landscape of great complexity. I always feel it is a wonder that we function on the whole as well as we do, with imbalance, we hope, the exception rather than the rule.

Margaret Thatcher

As I move from element to element I like to draw for each upon an example of a person in the public eye to illustrate the particular qualities which each reader is likely to be familiar with.* Since none of these are or have been my patients, for, if they were, professional ethics would prevent me from writing about them, my diagnosis is obviously taken from afar, based only upon those sensory and emotional signatures each display in photographs or on the television screen. Life as a famous person disperses many of the shadows within which each private person can hide themselves, and intense exposure to the spotlight of fame throws into sharper relief than normal many of the characteristics which define an element. We tend, however, to gain a very incomplete, distorted picture of those whose lives we glimpse only from the outside in this way, but because of this distortion this picture often highlights specific features of the elements which help us understand them better.

I have no personal experience of any of these people, except in the case of my example of the Earth element, Princess Diana, and my conclusions must always be qualified by the incomplete knowledge I have of each of them. I was fortunate enough to see her once as she passed my home on foot, and I can vouch

---

* The examples of famous people have been chosen primarily for British readers, but I hope they are also sufficiently well known to a wider audience.

for the astonishingly pure yellow of the colouring of her skin, which will be seen as evidence of Earth as we move on to discuss this element. With the very clear proviso, therefore, that my insights into the five famous people I have chosen must necessarily be incomplete, I offer you Margaret Thatcher as a further illustration of the Wood element.

What pointed me towards Wood in her case were above all her emotion and her voice. Both indicated that strong need for control which lies at the heart of Wood. And then there was that striking yet odd symbol which became a caricature of her power, the swinging handbag, bringing a touch of violence to this most feminine of all accessories, here turned into a weapon of aggression, its swing powerful enough to knock over those in her path. It was said that most of her cabinet ministers were frightened of her, expressing the fear of those forced regularly to confront anger. Her favourites were the people who stood up to her, which in acupuncture terms we would see as those able to offer her the clear boundaries within which she could be contained. She was happiest where force met force, as in the Falklands War, where Wood's ability to make quick decisions and its delight in confrontation came into play.

Her movements, too, were quick and decisive. She really did stride on to the field of action, as if every encounter was an engagement of some kind. And when she was eventually forced from power (and how much effort it required to get her to go!) I watched with interest to see how she would cope once all the edifices of power which accompany high office, all the busy day-to-day activities involving complex planning and decision-making, were suddenly taken from her, and she had to relinquish everything which supported the intense structure of her life. And she did not cope at all well in her retirement, apparently lost and ill at ease, unable to find a fresh purpose to her life, that new direction which Wood must find if it is to feel fulfilled. It was only when another structure was put in place for her, that of the lecture circuit, that she began to find her feet again. We could say that she had in effect been uprooted, for a while unable to see a future for herself.

In some ways she could be said to have had the vision which Wood needs to plan ahead, and yet in the debacle over the introduction of the Poll Tax, which was the start of her downfall, she was unable to see the repercussions of what she was doing, even though these were pointed out to her time and time again. Hers was indeed a blinkered vision in this respect, as she steadfastly stood by a plan and a decision made, unable to bring to them the flexibility Wood has to have to enable it to change and adapt to new situations when the need arises.

We can have no clearer evidence of Wood's shouting voice than hers, with its strident, ringing tone, its emphatic cadences, its quality of 'I will brook no refusal.' As a nation, we were indeed spoken to as though she was the parent and we the children who had to do her bidding. To some extent those who covet power on this scale always think that the path they wish the country to follow must be right one, but how this certainty of being in the right is conveyed to others may vary. If we compare Margaret Thatcher to Tony Blair, for instance, and we will see further on that he is an example of the Fire element, the kind of power they each wielded can be seen to differ. Both imposed a war upon this country, but in different ways. With the Falklands War there was no debate. The decision was made quickly and enforced equally quickly, with no concerted attempt either before or afterwards to justify the rights and wrongs of the decision.

With the Iraq War, on the other hand, there was an enormous amount of debate, however little this debate may have impacted upon a decision possibly taken well beforehand. There was much discussion, many appearances before the House of Commons and before the people both before and after the war to justify, and continue to justify, what Tony Blair felt was the right thing to do. This moral fervour, quite unlike Margaret Thatcher's more single-minded motivation, also stems from a belief that he is right and we are misguided if we do not agree with him, but unlike in Margaret Thatcher's case it leads him to try and convince us that what he is doing is morally right. This need to act on the basis of moral certainty requires some participation from us. He wants to communicate his reasoning to us and would like to convince us of its righteousness. Margaret Thatcher just told us what she was going to do, and was not bothered by public opinion in this way.

When we reach the Fire element, we will see that it always feels the need to communicate, to reach out to others. As illustration, watch Tony Blair's smile, a pure Fire smile which comes from the heart and lights up his face and warms those he smiles at so that they have to smile in reply. Compare this with a memory of Margaret Thatcher's smile, if you can even remember seeing her smile warmly. The warmth is lacking, and there is no attempt to draw us towards her.

Margaret Thatcher provides an excellent illustration of Wood's enjoyment in building a structure, here the government, within which to exercise control within firm boundaries. It gives us an example of an emotion which matches this, which we call by the name of anger, and a shouting voice through which this control is exercised.

My Wood mother

And now, closer to home, too, I have a further, more personal example before me. Over the years, we often build up our understanding of the elements by looking at those closest to us, our family and friends. And here I draw on an example of the Wood element which is very dear to me, for my growing library of pointers to this element was built up, among other things, from my observations of my mother. Whenever I think of Wood I am reminded always of her, with a pang of deep affection tinged with not a little exasperation, for my lifelong acquaintance with her provided me with deep insights into those qualities Wood imparts to those whose guardian element it is. And this element undoubtedly formed the dominant force in her life. One example of its action springs to mind, and always makes me smile when I think of it. It illustrates very neatly, I think, some more of this element's dominant characteristics.

A year or so before my mother's death at nearly 90, she rang to tell us all how desperately ill she was feeling and from different parts of London we converged on her house. To our surprise, she greeted us, not from her bed, but cheerfully from the top of the stairs, with great delight showing off a new dress she had just bought, for all the world like some little girl in her new party frock.

There are several reasons why this has remained for me a clear demonstration of the Wood element in action. I see many things at work which point to the Wood element within her as I look at the way she acted. She insisted first that we come immediately. Once we arrived, she showed no compunction at having disturbed our evening so apparently frivolously. She showed that she could change from despair to happiness as though a switch had been turned on and off. She was irritated because our mood did not match hers, expecting us to change from natural concern for her welfare to cheerfulness in a matter of minutes. She was completely unaware that we might view her behaviour as inappropriate in any way.

This incident showed a need to control (insisting that we come quickly), a lack of concern for others (Wood's need to concentrate its attention upon a single action), an ability to switch mood and an insistence that we should feel the same as she does. She showed other characteristics, too, which were the work of the other elements within her, for we are formed by all the elements, but the most striking features in this encounter with her were those pointing to the Wood element. Some of these features could be considered appropriate, others not. And it is upon often very fine distinctions as to whether something is appropriate or not that our judgement of what is balanced or not is based.

In nature, the Wood element has to show that it can control the abundant growth of spring to allow some buds to mature and blossom in summer, and others to wither and die. Its control must not be so harsh that all buds wither, nor so slack that growth is unconfined. Similarly, it is necessary for a part of us to insist upon our own rights even at the expense of others, just as we need to focus upon what we are doing without being too distracted by what is around us. We need to exercise these qualities in a way which allows others, too, the right to manoeuvre, much as one bud must allow another the space to stretch towards the sunlight. To remain in balance, the Wood element in us must have a similar ability to control its natural desire for action. Some of my mother's actions showed evidence of what could be considered an appropriate expression of the element during our evening with her, others less so. Where I consider that this tipped over into imbalance is a matter to some extent of my subjective judgement, and again it is experience which teaches me how accurate this judgement is.

Was it appropriate for my mother, at nearly 90, to take such a childlike or childish pleasure in showing us her new clothes in this way and so late at night? Was her indifference to the fact that she had put us to considerable inconvenience appropriate? To these questions part of the answer is yes and part no. Nothing is so black and white that we can put an action into a category clearly labelled totally one thing or another. What can be an appropriate, balanced reaction or way of behaving can tilt over surprisingly quickly into imbalance.

My mother's joy in the simple things of life, a feature of her character throughout her life, shown here by her pleasure in her frock, can be seen as delightful, and often was regarded as such by us, and only became irritating when she took no notice of how this pleasure might affect others. To act like a child when one is a child is appropriate. To act like a child when one is an adult is not. The picture of my mother standing happily in her new dress at the top of the stairs has something both of the childlike and the childish in it. It makes me smile as evidence of a delight in what could, viewed from the vantage point of her age, be called childish, but also a rare pleasure in life which all children have, until it is squeezed out of them as they grow older. Here this can be seen as both an appropriate and inappropriate expression of the Wood element. It is appropriate to enjoy life. It is inappropriate to be joyful at a time when others have been told by you that you are very ill.

My mother's demand that we drop everything for her sake shows an ability and a desire to control those around her. Reluctant though we all were to be drawn from our family hearths to her home late at night, yet we all did her bidding. And we had had numerous previous examples of her ability to demand our presence inappropriately to call upon. Once we had arrived, instead of sending us away again now that she felt fine, she continued to demand our attendance upon her. It was late before we could leave. In effect she had taken control of the situation and of us. She had got her way. Indeed, we felt our own roles were controlled by her, as she demanded we play the parts she laid down for us, being expected at one moment to show our deep concern for her, at the next to join in her delight. That evening we were disempowered, and to some extent this was true of many of our dealings with her, for she needed always to some extent to be in control of people, and who better to control than her family? Here, too, there was evidence of the appropriate level of control all Wood people need to exercise, in this instance that of a mother over her children, and an inappropriate level revealed by her need to dictate our enjoyment of the evening.

And the emotion her exertion of control evoked in us, and, when we demurred slightly at her insistence that we partake in her joy, was anger. We felt we had been called to her aid under false pretences, and this made us angry. She, too, was irritated by the fact that we could not match her enthusiasm. In fact, she had not pretended that she was ill, but like a child she needed immediate support from others to deal with what we realized later was just a brief period of feeling slightly unwell. The knowledge that we were coming made her feel immediately better and enabled her to dress up for us.

This ability to live in the moment, experiencing despair one minute, joy the next, is one that we all demonstrate as children. It is this which makes it possible for a child to run crying to its mother, ask her to 'kiss it better' and run away laughing as if nothing had happened. The Wood element, the child among the elements, with its desire for action, is impatient to get on with the next thing and will not wish to linger in any one state for long. It will therefore seek quick satisfactions and quick solutions to allow room for the next thing to take its place. Once my mother knew we were coming, she could move on from worry about how ill she felt to the need to welcome us.

Her ability to switch mood so suddenly demonstrates one of Wood's strengths, its ability to live in the moment and not linger too long on things. This is the exact reverse, we shall see, of the Metal element, whose favoured place of repose is the past. But here we see an inappropriate expression of this inconstancy of Wood. Certainly it did not match that of her family who remained for most of the evening somewhat shocked at the ease with which our mother had forgotten a level of distress which had drawn us so urgently to her.

My mother's behaviour that evening veered from one side of the spectrum which Wood can present to the other. What started off as an example of unbalanced Wood by the end of the evening had taken on the delightful qualities which made of my mother throughout her life an interesting and lively companion to many. By the time we left, our anger, too, had softened into the amused but affectionate sense of mild to severe irritation which she often aroused in us. Our initial feeling of disempowerment gradually diminished, and such is Wood's natural cheerfulness and power that we were pulled in my mother's wake, almost against our will, into enjoying the dress show she presented us with so unexpectedly, seeing it for what it was, a somewhat inappropriate and yet at heart innocent delight in simple pleasures, a quality in her which never withered.

The manipulations we felt we had been a party to to get us to her side could now be seen for what they were, my mother's way of ensuring that she wasn't left alone for too long. The feelings of distress with which she called us were real, just as the speed of her recovery was real. To that extent she was as much the victim of the need for control as we were.

It will now be interesting to compare the similarities and differences between two of the Wood people we have looked at so far, my mother and James, who I used as an example of how we start our interactions with a patient. This will add a further layer to our understanding of this element.

Both have a natural vivacity, an eagerness to get on with things, an ability to live in the moment, a quickness of humour as well as of temper, a natural aggression, often a little bit unbridled, and a need for control. They both show evidence of that push, the clenched fist, the determination to get on with things, which I have shown to be one of Wood's characteristics. They both, too, respond well to boundaries drawn by others who are in a position of control, and they have a quality of exuberant energy reflecting that of spring. Diagnostically, too, they have a similar timbre to their voices, a similar smell upon them, very familiar to me from my years with my mother, and a similar greenish tint to their skin. They both easily show their irritation when things do not go their way.

But my diagnosis cannot stop here, for both are unique emanations of this energy, with needs of their own which differ from each other's, and requiring treatment specifically geared to these needs. They occupy their own particular place within the territory which Wood occupies, each of them forming a tiny facet of that vast whole we call the energy of a particular element, just as each bud on a tree, apparently springing from the same source, is uniquely shaped, and, if allowed to flourish and eventually seed itself, will create a tree uniquely different from any other tree of its species.

If we look at Wood manifesting in nature, we can see it showing many faces. It creates the roots from which all plants emerge, the trunks which these roots support and the branches they grow their leaves upon. It takes many shapes. Pliant, it can be used to sweep the floor, and can be shaped into baskets or wickerwork. Its firm contours can be cut and moulded to create toys, bowls and furniture. It is caressing to the touch, for there remains in everything wooden always something of the living sap which created it, giving to what the carpenter shapes that feeling of a still living thing. It can be supple as willow, delicate as bamboo or inflexible as oak. It is the tender stalk of a daffodil and the tough shell of a walnut. It can be dry as tinder, the merest glint of sun upon a sliver of glass turning it into the flames which feed a forest fire. It can soften or rot, as the daffodil's stalk will rot if standing in too much water. It can shrivel, as the walnut's shell will do once its sap dries up.

The different qualities of all these aspects of Wood are imparted to it by some of the qualities of the other elements. Where the daffodil rots it is because its roots are drowned in Water. Where the walnut shell dries up, it is because the air in which it lives (Metal) is not fed sufficiently by its sap (Wood). Thus we say that one person's Wood element might have a lot of Fire or Water in it, for example. If it is a fiery Wood, the green colour is tinged with a slight hint of red, the anger with a slight hint of Fire's joy. If it is a watery Wood, the colour will be tinged with blue, the anger with fear.

James' Wood element contains a strong hint of Metal within it, giving his anger the cutting edge which we will see grief, Metal's emotion, can add to things, and laying a whiteish tinge on the green on his skin. The shouting voice has a slightly sad tone to it and his smell has some of the autumn smell we associate with Metal. Buried inside my mother's Wood, on the other hand, was a quite different need, that of a cry for sympathy, the domain of Earth. This tinge of the Earth element within her Wood gave her colour a yellowish-green tone, added a lilt to her shouting voice and some of the sweet smell of Earth to her underlying Wood smell. While both have a need for order and control, in my mother's case this was modified by a strong appeal for others to look after her, as the incident I described shows. James, on the other hand, demands that those around him give him some of the space Metal always seeks.

Each of the many nuances which differentiate one person from another within the same element is therefore created by some slight modification of this element by qualities brought to it from the other elements. A painter asked to select the right pigment to illustrate the colours on their skin would thus select different shades of green for James and my mother. A musician would hear different tones in their shouting voices. Emotionally, their approach to life differs slightly. But these differences are always contained, just as colour, sound and smell are, within the boundaries of what we have seen to be the territory in which the Wood element operates.

These sensory messages are not fixed as though written on stone. They are fluid, as the elements which convey them reflect the ever-changing movement inherent in all things. A patient's expression of anger may be exaggerated in spring, or modified by the action of other elements upon it, and thus diagnosis and treatment will reflect the changing landscape through which the patient moves from day to day and year to year. A treatment selected today cannot therefore be repeated tomorrow.

CHAPTER 6

THE FIRE ELEMENT

With a pang of regret I leave my mother, for our journey now leads us in another direction, on to Fire, the child of Wood, and to the territory of my own element, making me, like the seasons which we reflect, a Fire child to my mother's Wood. The dial of the elements has turned on a little further, pointing me to the south and to a landscape filled with sunlight. So into summer, Fire's season, we now move, to find some understanding within nature of what this quality lends to those born under Fire's patronage.

It is early summer now. I am walking along paths I walked along some weeks ago. Where before I saw clearly ahead, now my way is blocked by tendrils of bushes, blackberry and nettle which snake across from side to side, catching at my feet and forcing me to push my way through. All the growing things around me which only a little while ago were mere bursts of activity on twig and bough are now fully swollen, their branching arms in their profusion reaching out, blocking my way and closing down the horizon. Much is now lost to view behind all this growth. The far horizon, visible in winter through the bare branches of trees and punctuated in spring by the sharp outlines of the buds, is now crowded out by all this abundant new life. As I look around I see an entirely new landscape. The energetic explosion of spring has calmed down into a more gentle unfolding. There is a fullness to all things, an abundance, a stretching out to its fullest extent, as though arms are flung wide to the sky above and around me. Here I walk surrounded on all sides, in the midst of nature's greatest, most visible offering, as though enfolded.

The summer landscape spreads up far above my head and to right and left of me, profuse and yet, at human height, close, blocking my view to all but what is around me. I can see today the paradox which lies at the heart of Fire, as it does of each element. This most open of all elements has its horizon limited by the abundance of growth around it. Surprisingly for an element of such insight, as we will see later, Fire's vision here appears to be the most limited of all, hampered on all sides by what is around it which prevents it from seeing the long view.

Today the sun weighs heavily upon me. It is exceptionally hot for early summer, with spring only just disappearing round the corner, and this heat challenges me, doesn't let me be, makes me clammy and lethargic. So much heat so soon seems to have caught me unawares, pushing me out into the sunlight before I was ready. There is a greater languor in the air. Some of the moisture of the sap has gone, drying things out. I, too, feel heavy in the heat, dried out, my feet dragging a little, my eyes squinting against the sun. What is this force that has the strength to push all nature out to its furthest extent and yet weighs upon me? Here, observed in nature, Fire is not a light element, and its thrust, like that of Wood, is strong.

Yesterday the sun shone, lighting up much of the overgrown paths and laying a dappling of bright colour over all things, but today all is gloom, all its brightness hidden behind lowering clouds. And where what was clear, all now seems to be shadowed and overcast, so that as I walk under the trees I feel oppressed, their shades not comforting as yesterday's were, but slightly threatening. I am made aware of the sharp contrasts which this dull day evokes in me. Where before I felt open, outward-looking, happy, today I feel a weight upon me. There are darker shadows under the trees in the gloom of a sunlit summer's day than at any other time of the year. Nature appears in starker contrasts, more black and white, the extremes of light and brightness the sun offers us counterbalanced by the shadows leaf and blossom spread under them when clouds cover them. We become for a moment blinded as we walk out of the sun under the trees, and, as we move into this darkness, nature can feel quite threatening until our eyes regain their sight.

There is an expectation of the sun's presence throughout our summers, and then a disappointment when it fails to appear. We experience a lack of something that should be there that is not, a feeling no other season evokes in quite the same way, for to none but summer does the sun bestow the full span of a day's sunshine, shedding the brightest, hottest light upon things. The other elements demand different things of the sun's heat. Wood delights in a freshness to its warmth, Earth basks in its afterglow, whilst Metal welcomes the coolness of autumn and Water the cold of the winter sun. To none but summer is the strength of the sun's heat a dominating need, and when the sun is hidden, for however brief a time, as it is on this dull day, its partial presence, after all yesterday's abundant warmth, shocks and disappoints me. I feel strangely cast down, overcast as is the sky, as that exhilarating expansion under the sun which I experienced yesterday is blotted out as though a hand has been placed over the sun, and with it a hand over my heart.

Such indeed are the contrasts this most volatile of all elements has to live with, the bright sunlight as the Heart, our own sun within us, sings with joy, dark shadows as this sun is hidden and our Heart becomes oppressed. This reflects the pressures the Fire element experiences as we move from light to shade in our relationships with others, for we will see that Fire is concerned above all with the nature of these relationships. The time of childhood and early youth represented by the element Wood now passes, with summer, into the time of the young adult, as we move out into the wider world and find our place within it. The bud becomes aware of those other buds surrounding it on the bough.

With Fire we move into the demanding world of the other. Having grown beyond our pressing need to ensure our own existence, which is Wood's task, we now turn our face towards what surrounds us, finding our interest now in exploring the nature of how we interact with that strange, exhilarating but often threatening world inhabited by those amongst whom we live. This is a demanding task, for it asks of us that we learn to affirm our right to be ourselves whilst accepting that others, too, have a similar right.

No longer content with our own company, we move, with Fire, out of childhood, out of the time of the new and unformed, into that of emerging adulthood, which brings with it the start of our responsibilities to those with whom we are to spend the remainder of our lives, our family, friends, partners, workmates and that great mass of still unknown strangers to whom it is Fire's task to attempt, in many different ways, to stretch out arms of welcome. For the contact of one being with another, and the dramas which play themselves out in terms of human relationships, are the stage on which it is at home. It may shrink from the spotlight, fearing sometimes too bright a glare, but it cannot remove itself from the play, for it is intimately involved in all the subtle manoeuvrings we engage in when we encounter another human being.

Just as the blossom slowly unravels itself from the bud, so does our true nature as an independent human being unique in need and character begin to unfold, tempered by our interactions with others. Those skirmishes often deeply felt, as we align and realign ourselves with new friends in the school playground and discard the old, and then move slowly on to our first sexual encounters, these all form part of the development of ourselves as we start to be more independent of the tight hold our families have upon us. All of those we rub up against round off or sharpen our edges as we learn to delineate our own boundaries. It is the Fire element which guides us amidst this profusion of activity.

Where Wood is there to give us hope, Fire, above all, bestows love and joy, and those with Fire as their guardian element can no more shed the rosy-coloured spectacles of love which this element forces us to look through than those sheltering under Wood's umbrella can throw off their need to get out there and get things going. Joy is the air that Fire breathes, where Wood breathes action. And its voice, so important to Fire as one of its instruments of communication, in its tones carries laughter, the welcoming sound of joy. Even when Fire's loving is buffeted by blows, and laughter fades from it, faint traces can still be heard, often breaking out inappropriately where laughter there should be none. This is Fire's way of keeping its Heart warm, for if the storms of life blow angrily against it, it will attempt to stoke up a small bonfire of joy by laughing at itself. And the smell of such bonfires, a scorched, hot smell, will be the smell of Fire.

The Heart has potentially unlimited stores of love to offer and an unlimited number of recipients upon whom to bestow this love. Each encounter with another can become a tiny act of transformation, offering the possibility of making both of us in this partnership a little different and a little more than we were before we met each other. The field of love stretches on all sides further than the eye can see or arm can reach, and such a potential number of transformations is as limitless as the number of people available for us to meet. To Fire people, whose Heart wishes to offer itself to all, this fusion of themselves with others, seen symbolically through the reaching out of their smiles and their laughter, is the arena upon which they must act out their life. Talk to a Wood person, and you will hear discussion of actions, of things to be done, of an eagerness to get on and do them. With Fire, on the other hand, the talk will be of people. The need to do is replaced by the need to include others in those actions.

And this very need to find other people to whom to relate makes it move out beyond itself into that often dangerous world where others have their being. Love is one of the most profound ways of entering the unknown world of others, and there is something courageous about all the attempts we make throughout our life to break beyond the safe confines of ourselves and reach out to those around us. These others can seem frighteningly not ourselves, turning all our relationships into so many attempts to bridge that almost unbridgeable gap between ourselves and others. It might indeed be safer to stay cocooned within the familiar boundaries of ourselves, but it is precisely this secure world which it is Fire's task to disrupt, for in its attempts to throw arms of love around as much of the world and its people as it can encompass in its grasp, it has to be prepared to move out beyond itself. And the word courage has the Latin word for heart buried deep within it, and the Heart is the ruler of Fire's domain.

In giving so much, its need is always to have someone there to give to, and this need for others makes it vulnerable. When its energy falters, this can translate into its two weaknesses, an exaggerated form of self-abnegation, being a denial of its own needs, or an inability to express its generosity for fear of being hurt. If we are prepared to open our hearts to love, we must be prepared not only to be welcomed but to be rebuffed and hurt. Exposing its flank thus widely to attack is one of the risks that Fire takes. Of all the elements, it is the one that is prepared to risk the most. Throwing off its clothes to greet the heat of the midsummer sun, Fire stands there as though naked before the gaze of all. It is the only element not ashamed of such openness, and is often surprisingly ready to reveal its own inadequacies and failures, believing such honesty is necessary to draw it closer to others.

All Fire does is at heart an act of communication and communion. Other elements, which prefer to burrow down rather than blaze out into the light, may look disapprovingly at Fire's great need to communicate so openly. To such elements, silence might indeed seem golden, but to Fire speech is golden, shedding warm sunlight upon all with its words.

A smile, symbol of Fire's capacity to offer love, becomes then a token of welcome we throw out to another, as we reach out to all we encounter and seek to understand the nature of these encounters, each smile a question-mark demanding an answer. There are as many smiles as there are differing relationships, and each will have a different purpose, come from a different place in our Heart and be received in differing ways by those we smile at. All of us, except the most disturbed or unhappy, can smile at times, whatever our element, because we all wish to relate to others in some way or other, but the nature of a smile will reflect the particular element whose messenger it is. In the case of the two elements we have looked at so far, the smiles will reveal different things. My mother smiling at the top of her stairs did not warm us, far from it. Her smile was not concerned with ensuring we were alright. It was her way of showing that she was. It had a more selfish cause, directed at her own satisfaction, and indicating that all was well for her. Fire's smile is quite different, for it is evidence of a concern for others, not for itself, to the extent that it will smile even when ill at ease, because it wishes not to disturb others with its unhappiness.

We can gauge the level of balance of a person's Fire element by the appropriate or inappropriate level of its need to reach out to others, indicated by this smile among things. If this need is excessive and out of proportion to what is required, it overshadows the person's ability to protect themselves. The smile will then appear at times which least call for smiling, such as when a person is talking about emotional distress and laughs, or when a person attempts to defuse another's anger by smiling too much.

Watch the rebuffs we experience when a smile we offer, and with it a tiny parcel of love, meets with no response. Feel how this chills our Heart, as though the sun has for a moment hidden behind clouds. Imagine the sadness of a life lived among relationships which never emerge from behind such clouds, where the sun of love is never allowed to shine. This is the area of hurt to which the Fire element within us and those of us with Fire as our guardian element are exposed and where its imbalances will lie.

Many of the problems Fire labours under are those caused by its own inability to deal appropriately with the myriad relationships it seeks to set up. When it is in balance it learns to shun those relationships which fan it to a fiery furnace, for if it burns out of control, anybody approaching it will indeed be playing with fire. It should burn steadily and truly, a pure flame warming those it approaches, feeding itself when it dies down too low, or restraining itself when it feels itself blazing forth. The need to sort relationships out, get them on an even keel and ensure that our defences are sufficiently strong to prevent hurt to the Heart is Fire's field of action. A delicate balance has to be drawn between openness, which brings vulnerability in its wake, and a closed heart which may lead us to reject others.

Fire's great gift is the bestowal of love. Fire's fear is that it will be prevented from reaching out to others to bestow this love. Fire's great learning is detachment. It has to learn to allow others the right to refuse its love, and remain undevastated by their refusal. It has to learn that it is safe to move around in a world where not everyone wants its love. It has to learn that there is a time not to love as well as a time to love.

The two sides of Fire

Unlike the other elements, the Fire element has a dual role, making it almost two elements twinned within one. It, too, is formed of two organs, here the Heart and Small Intestine, but it has two further aspects which spread their influence far more diffusely throughout body and soul. These are our blood circulation system and heat regulatory mechanisms, and are known in five element acupuncture by the names of the Heart Protector and Three Heater officials, though given other names in other traditions. Uniquely, even their names, let alone their functions, are shrouded in mystery and much debated, with some branches of acupuncture seeing in them one thing, others quite another. They are addressed much more directly in five element acupuncture than they are in other branches of acupuncture, perhaps because the official they are there to protect, the Heart, the ultimate controller of blood and heat, takes up such a dominant position in our tradition.

I call the organ pairing Inner Fire, the two functions Outer Fire, with the Inner Fire officials forming a nucleus around which the Three Heater and Heart Protector officials spread their protective arms. Both aspects of Fire have in common its specific sensory characteristics, imprinted upon them in a red colouring, a laughing voice, a scorched smell and the expression of the emotion we call joy in its many aspects. And it is in the last, in their emotional orientation to life, that we can begin to pinpoint some of the differences between the two aspects which lend a distinctive shading to those under Fire's protection, orientate them differently to the world and require a different focus to their treatments.

The function of both aspects in their differing ways is to protect the Heart in their midst. Acupuncturists regard it as the lord and emperor of the kingdom of body and soul, selflessly watching over this kingdom. It bears full responsibility for all that happens within its domain, sending constant messengers along the great highways of the blood to the furthest outposts of its kingdom to ensure that all the other organs function as they should. The steady throb of our heartbeat pulsing throughout every channel of our body announces its watchful presence, and, like some watchman of the night sounding the hours, assures us that all is well. And it must work tirelessly, for if its attention slackens however briefly, shudders of distress will echo throughout its kingdom, the merest flutter or hesitation in our heartbeat causing us panic and fear. It seems to do so little, hidden from sight deep within us, and yet all is dependent upon its strength.

The pathways of energy which acupuncture recognizes as the Fire meridians include within their sphere of protection the physical organ of the heart as well as its deeper manifestations, which we all recognize in everyday speech as we admit to being broken-hearted, or warm to those who are kind-hearted. When we chide one another for being cold-hearted, we do not visualize our physical heart growing cold to the touch, nor do we imagine this heart's temperature rising as our heart is warmed by others' kindnesses. It is this more profound and all-encompassing concept to which the Chinese gave the name of Heart, and which acupuncturists approach with awe, for it is upon its bounty and health that each of our lives depends. It is considered a sacred organ, and in some traditions is never treated.

The physical heart lies hidden within our chest, protected at the front by the muscle and bone of the pericardium and ribs, and at the back by the heavy fortifications of the vertebrae and backbone. It is also protected by the two wings of the lungs which enfold it. Chinese medicine also recognizes that the official we call the Heart is given a further protective framework in the two Outer Fire officials, and it is to this outer periphery of Fire that I now turn to help us understand the nature of the Fire element a little more deeply.

The Three Heater and the Heart Protector form an odd pairing within the family of officials, unattached directly to any organ but allied to the Heart and Small Intestine as they shelter within the Fire element. They have the widest remit of all the officials, their territory extending throughout every part of the body and soul, the one maintaining life-giving warmth, the other maintaining life-giving blood. Both can be seen as forming the ramparts of the Heart's castle, an outer line of defence enclosing the Heart in their midst and providing a protective barrier to hold the world at bay.

Outer Fire represents the face Fire turns to the outside world, its acceptable, smiling face, the one that is there to form a bridge to others beyond it. Being open to the outside, it is very much influenced by external pressures upon it, physically represented by the adjustments in temperature and blood flow we have to make all the time to remain alive. It can be seen as Fire's more sociable side, concerned with smoothing the interrelationships with others demanded of us by the need to integrate ourselves within a social framework. It is the face we probably conjure up first when we think of the words joy and love. In acupuncture terms, Outer Fire's task, through the differing activities of its two officials, is to maintain the outer defensive network behind which the Heart can be sheltered, and thus it is concerned with ensuring that any relationships entered into are first approached with caution. Strong Outer Fire defences are those which warn us to avoid a friend who is sarcastic to us, a workmate who criticizes us or a partner who makes us uneasy, before any of these have had the chance so to breach the Heart's defences as to damage it deeply or even irrevocably. The Outer Fire officials can therefore be regarded symbolically as guards patrolling the Heart's ramparts, warning the Heart if somebody approaching it is unsafe for it to relate to.

With Inner Fire, and the Heart itself, we enter another, more hidden domain. And here we move inside to Fire's more inward-looking side, guarded by the Small Intestine, the last of the Heart's protectors. In Western medicine one of the small intestine's function is to sift the products the stomach has processed, extract from them the good nutrients, and pass these through the walls of the blood vessels into the bloodstream to feed the heart. In Chinese medicine, to this physical function is added that deeper level which all officials possess. It is regarded not only as allowing through to the Heart only what is pure in the form of blood, but as having the wider remit all officials have of protecting the Heart at an emotional level, too, sifting what approaches it, as it does physically to the blood, and discarding to the Large Intestine what it judges to be waste material. Whereas a strong Heart Protector and Three Heater ensure that the Heart can make its judgements safely and without fear of attack, a strong Small Intestine ensures that these judgements are wise.

Inner Fire's role is concerned with the important matters of life and death over which the Heart resides, for it has to get things right for the whole kingdom of body and soul, and thus this axis of Fire turns a much more serious face to the world than does its Outer Fire counterpart. Indeed, we may even have some difficulty in seeing people who are related to the inner aspect of Fire as residing within the Fire element at all, since they often lack some of the obvious expressions of joy and laughter which we think of as Fire's rightful domain, apparently having little time for the more bubbly, overt expressions of happiness which Outer Fire can take such pleasure in.

The Small Intestine in its role as efficient secretary to the Heart has the responsibility of ensuring that it advises the Heart and all the other officials wisely. This requires sustained, hard work. It will ponder long over what is the right thing for the Heart to do, and will constantly be exercised by a concern that its actions are appropriate. It regards life as a puzzle to be unravelled, a series of constant question marks to which it has to find the correct answers. You see on its face often a querying look, a slightly wrinkled brow, as it listens to what you are saying and then puts the cogs of its mind into motion to make sense of what it hears. An Inner Fire person makes an excellent jigsaw puzzler, able to see connections more quickly than others, visually and orally perceptive to the slightest nuance. It is by far the most naturally quick-witted of all the officials, for it has rapidly to unravel a coherent pattern from what comes towards it so that it has time to advise the Heart how to act.

Billy Connolly and Tony Blair

To help illustrate these two aspects of Fire further, I will now conjure up the comedian Billy Connolly before us, for I can find no better example of the outer aspect of the Fire element in action than this. And as I think of him now, I feel a reflection of the warm glow in which he enveloped me and all his TV audience one evening some months ago. He stood alone on the stage and yet he stretched out to everyone out there in the theatre and beyond them to the millions watching. As we laughed with him, we became at one with him and with each other, bathed in joy for the span of the performance. Even now, when I think back to this performance a long time ago, I start to smile although I am not quite sure what I am smiling at. I can't remember what he was talking about, but I experience again traces of the feeling of happiness he gave me then. There is no better testimonial to the capacity of Outer Fire to bring warmth and joy to us.

What does he do to make us feel so close to him? He seems to be reaching out to every one of us, drawing us towards him by making us laugh. The candour with which he tells us about his deepest feelings reflects a trust in us which makes us feel close to him. He comes towards us his arms open to greet us and lays himself bare before us. He does not seek to hide what is in his heart, whether it be pain or joy, and he makes no attempt to cover up his own weaknesses and inadequacies. Indeed, they form the central theme of all he talks about. Here is the courage which is a hallmark of Fire, for in exposing his inner being to the public gaze of millions he can be seen as making himself vulnerable. And who but he knows how much such a performance may take out of him? Potentially he is risking a great deal, but this he is prepared to do because such openness is necessary if he wishes to enter into the close relationships with us which makes each of us his intimate friend. We do not have time to abuse the trust he puts in us, before the relationship he sets up with us makes this impossible.

In effect, he is saying 'Look at me and the people I talk to you about in all our pettiness and stupidity and inadequacy.

Am I not ridiculous, and is not life ridiculous? I need to share all this hurt and pain with you out there, and together we have to see things for what they are and learn to laugh at fate.' And in thus offering himself to us so openly, he engages with us at our deepest level, as we see reflected in him our own pettinesses, stupidities and inadequacies. Above all, he shows us by example the importance of our relationships with one another, here symbolized by his warm contact with us. Listen to him, and no sentence is complete without reference to a person, either to himself or to others, and then a reference to the audience so that all are drawn together.

The acuteness of ear and eye which he brings to bear on all his encounters so that he can evoke a human situation in a few words in all its complexity is evidence of Fire's awareness of people, its understanding of their interactions with one another and the importance it feels in seeing things as they are. The laughing voice, the red colour and the emotion of joy flood out from our TV screens, bathing us in warmth. This is Outer Fire truly in its element, but in exaggerated form, as befits the heightened level of experience demanded by a performance such as this. If we were to continue to live at this level beyond the few hours we are with him, the intensity of this encounter would start to shrivel both performer and audience. This is an example of what might happen if Fire is stoked up too high for too long, burning itself and others out. It also has to know how to flicker softly and low to recharge its batteries.

Does Billy Connolly laugh too much? Would we be uneasy with all this warmth in our everyday life? These, and many other similar questions, are good things to ask to help us determine what we can consider the balanced or unbalanced aspects of the manifestations of the Outer Fire officials. All comedians to a greater or lesser extent must draw upon the Fire in themselves and in their audience to raise the laughter which is a measure of their success. Each performance is then a re-affirmation of our delight in the contacts we can make with one another. I have used Billy Connolly's stage presence as a very vivid example of Outer Fire's power to reach out to others, and to illustrate Fire's face turned, very publicly in this example, to the outside world. As an example of the Outer Fire officials burning bright this cannot be equalled.

For an example of Inner Fire I turn now to Tony Blair, and as I think of him, I experience a slight jolt, as though I am taken slightly aback at the idea of placing him and Billy Connolly within the same elemental territory. There is something so open about Billy Connolly, and something much more closed and hidden about Tony Blair, so how can they both be seen as being of the same element? When I look carefully at the reasons for my unease, I realize that in my instinctive reaction lies something which will help me describe something of the nature of the essential difference which enable us to pinpoint one or other side of Fire.

I think first of Tony Blair's smile as he beamed his welcome to a visitor to Downing Street. Billy Connolly's smile evokes a much more open, immediate response from me, which chimes more easily with the atmosphere of joy and laughter he spreads around him. Blair, on the other hand, brings with him a seriousness of manner broken into by his very warm smile, and then returning to a more serious mode once the smile has gone. It is as though the sun comes out for a moment, and then retreats behind clouds again. In acupuncture terms, the Inner Fire officials, with the Heart at their midst, are always aware of the gravity of what they do in terms of keeping us alive, and return to this gravity once the moment of interaction with others has passed.

Symbolically, Tony Blair would no doubt have seen his role as Prime Minister as having kept this country functioning, a somewhat surprisingly apt metaphor for the role of the Inner Fire officials within us. Like our physical heart, which relies upon other organs to provide it with the energy to keep us functioning, he, too, needed to work with a band of close allies who help him, each in their differing ways reflecting some aspect of the role of the Small Intestine official. For it is this official's task to sift and sort and discard whatever reaches Fire's inner periphery, before it is considered appropriate to pass it on to the Heart, as final arbiter of what is right for the kingdom of body and soul. I have often thought that this may well be one of the reasons why he needed to surround himself with powerful aides, chief among them Peter Mandelson who took on this role in many guises throughout Blair's tenure in Downing Street. This may help to explain his constant re-emergence in transformed guise, for he offered something which appeared to be essential to Blair and which is often puzzling to others.

In acupuncture terms the Heart, a yin organ, needs its yang companion to do all the hard work behind the scenes, advising the Heart to accept only what is pure and discarding what it is not right to retain. This is also the role our physical small intestine plays, an example of how closely the Chinese concept of the body mirrors its Western counterpart at many levels. On the larger stage of politics, Blair's band of advisers fulfilled a similar function, acting as a secretariat through whose offices all must pass to reach the Prime Minister. Blair always proved heavily reliant on their advice, often, to the outside eye, disturbingly so. They worked mostly behind the scenes, and were therefore all the more threatening to others for acting out such hidden roles, which may explain the antagonism aroused by people such Peter Mandelson and Alastair Campbell, another powerful aide. In their differing ways, and in different transformations over the years, these two in particular have acted as private secretaries to whom Blair turned to provide him with what he obviously regarded as sound advice and insights into what was going on around him.

I have always found it interesting to see how such an apparently strong person as Blair had needed to surround himself with a team of equally strong helpers, whose strength, far from being threatening to him, he appeared to welcome, whereas Margaret Thatcher, another strong person, in a similar position needed very few advisers around her, choosing instead to make her own mind up about things, and often dismissing those who challenged her. The role of Blair to Mandelson reflected the good relationship which should exist between the Heart and Small Intestine, mutually dependent and mutually supportive of each other, the Small Intestine deferring always to the Heart's pre-eminence, and the Heart secure enough in its dominant position to welcome to itself what it judges to be the strength and wisdom of others.

Tony Blair showed other qualities which help us illustrate the workings of Inner Fire. He showed that he needed to listen to others, but not necessarily be swayed by them, finally being quite secure in his own decisions, as strikingly shown in what can be regarded as his stubbornness in relation to his decision to go to war in Iraq. He is imbued with a kind of moral fervour, and however warily we may view this, it undoubtedly stems from a pure conviction emanating from his Heart that he is doing right, one of Inner Fire's greatest challenges. For not to do right is what Inner Fire regards not only as a failure but as morally indefensible, for it sees this as leading to a loss of direction and even to corruption in the kingdom of the body and soul, for it regards a kingdom bereft of good leadership as moving on the path to anarchy.

In all the actions Inner Fire takes there is an echo of the tension within the constant activity of the physical small intestine in its efforts to purify all that comes through to it from the stomach, and some of this restless tension is visible in Tony Blair's body and speech. His quick movements give an impression of pent-up energy, far removed from the more relaxed movements of Billy Connolly. Tony Blair walking into a press conference appears to be throwing out a challenge to the press, whereas Billy Connolly walking on to the stage welcomes us. Listen, too, to Tony Blair's voice, as he talks from the heart, passionate, convincing, but often, too, struggling to find exactly the right word to express this passion, this need to say what he regards it as his duty to express, and thus stumbling a little on himself, as his mind, such an active part of Inner Fire, tries first to look this way and then that before replying to a question, so important is it to Inner Fire that it gets the answers right.

Compare this rather more uneven speech with the articulate, but equally impassioned speech of Billy Connolly. And however manic he may appear, there is something much more mellow and less driven about Billy Connolly's movements on stage than there is about Tony Blair's whole demeanour. I would guess that most of us would prefer to spend a few hours in Billy Connolly's company rather than Tony Blair's for this reason. I see this as an example of Outer Fire's task to look to our comfort and well-being, and its ability to relax, once it is sure that we are comfortable and safe. Inner Fire, more driven and striving always for the good of the kingdom, remains restless in its quest to unravel the puzzles of life and find answers for the Heart, and causes us to feel slightly restless and uneasy in its presence, as though we, too, like the Heart, pulsing steadily from birth to death, can never be quite at rest in its presence.

A Fire patient

I have chosen a further illustration of Outer Fire from my practice. My patient, Rebecca, illustrates for me some of those qualities we saw as being characteristic of this aspect of Fire – warmth, enjoyment in personal contact, a sense of fun, allied to, deep within, a vulnerability, that sense of exposure to the potential rejection of all these offerings to others which Outer Fire is so determined to make.

She is a young woman of 25, a gifted musician with the world at her feet, and yet she is beset by self-doubt and feelings of inadequacy. She came for treatment initially for help with shoulder pain. As a flautist, she was concerned that the physical discomfort she was suffering from was beginning to affect the strength of the arm which bore the weight of the flute. Though she started by telling me about her shoulder pain, very soon I found myself instead listening to an impassioned discussion of all the people in her life. I discovered that she had a history of unhappy friendships, and a series of sexual relationships none of which had lasted longer than a few months. It was her interest in discussing her interactions with others, not her physical complaints, which absorbed all our time together, and continues to do so to a strikingly greater extent than occurs when I am with other non-Fire patients. People and her relations to them are her abiding concern. The pain in her shoulders, though threatening her professional life, has never been as central to her concerns as are the perturbed waters of her relationships. There is here a clear focus to her life and it leads directly away from herself to other people.

She always feels it is her responsibility to get these relationships right, working away at them energetically to try to help them gain some of the purity and honesty which the Heart requires if it is to love deeply. She struggles to make her relationships work, and is concerned to smooth the path of others through life, trying to ensure that in whatever situation she finds herself those around her are alright, even to the detriment of her own needs. She offers herself, in smiles, words and deeds, in an attempt to bring that joy to others which is her own emotional resting place.

When she first came for treatment, her imbalance expressed itself as a sense of deep vulnerability. It was as though she had no energy to maintain the defences her Outer Fire officials offered the Heart to enable her to stand back and assess her relationships with others properly. She had a tendency either to open herself up too quickly and unwisely to others around her or to close herself off from them when such openness led to hurt. This explained the speed at which she ended her sexual explorations, and the turbulent nature of some of her friendships. She seemed to jump into each new relationship, sexual or otherwise, as though with her eyes shut, too afraid to look.

It was interesting to see how her posture had taken on some of the vulnerability she showed emotionally, and I felt this went some way to explaining why she had such bad shoulder pains. Her back was hunched, her neck muscles tight, and she often clasped her arms tightly in front of her in an instinctive gesture of defence. As her treatment progressed, her strengthened Outer Fire officials enabled her to protect herself better and she became increasingly secure within herself. She began to see that to look before she jumped was a sensible and necessary first step in any new encounter. I was interested to note how cautious she became as she started to gauge whether a person she met was going to add to her life or bring problems, was in fact safe to approach. I felt treatment had been successful when she reported one day triumphantly that she felt somebody she had just met wasn't the right sort of person for her to go out with. I saw this as evidence that Fire's defensive network was now strong enough to shelter her from damage, and was providing her with the necessary protection to enable her Heart, with the Small Intestine's help, to judge appropriately what she should do.

All these changes impacted directly upon her physical posture. She no longer clenched her arms so tightly to her and walked more upright, with her shoulders thrown back. Her neck muscles relaxed, and in turn so did those of her jaw. She told me that she had had to go back to her teacher for further lessons to readjust her flute position because of these changes in posture! I interpreted this as a sign that her internal defence mechanisms were sufficiently strong not to need to draw on the physical reserves of her arms to protect her. All these changes reduced her worries about the future of her professional work whilst adding to the appearance she gave of being more open to others and more confident in herself.

If, now, we are to compare my patient Rebecca to James, my Wood patient, we would say that James lives his life much more towards the outside, in the successful completion of his daily routines, whilst Rebecca lives more towards the inside, in the more complex world of relationships. When reading my description of her, I also note the absence of any references to the complex dynamics between the two of us with which my description of my interaction with James is peppered. The area of difficulty lies not in the relationship between us and the element of power struggle I described with James as we worked out the boundaries between us, but in shoring up Rebecca's sensitivity to the intrusions of others.

She is only compliant as far as she judges my comments and assessments of any situation to be accurate. Although she actively welcomes my participation and guidance, she closes herself off if I err on the side of what she thinks is too strong an interference, in effect closing her Heart to me and putting up an impenetrable wall. This is a protective mechanism, and shows its imbalance by an excessive need to overprotect itself, much as James' Wood element will show an excessive need for control. This is an illustration of her tendency, curbed but not totally eliminated by the balance brought to her through her treatment, to misinterpret approaches made by others because of what can become an unbalanced assessment of the nature of the relationships she enters into.

Fire under pressure
The relationships of one human being to another introduce areas of conflict which no animal, made apparently of simpler stuff and needing simpler things from its relationships with its fellows, is prone to. Just as the complexity of the human body leads to complexity of operation compared with that of the more advanced animal species, and thus increased scope for

breakdown, so the complexity of our emotional and spiritual life places similarly increased demands upon each one of us. It is little wonder, then, given this, that that most sacred and special part of us, over which our Heart rules, is also the area of our greatest stresses. The Fire element is called upon to work at its busiest when we rub up against each other in an increasingly complex world where our relationships with each other extend far beyond the small and intimate circle of the primitive village lost in the jungle.

We need only look at our TV screen each day for evidence of this. Here we see vast audiences of people, both at home and in the studio, drawn into a web of different relationships, as the world of chat show, Big Brother, X Factor and similar types of programme, more and more unscrupulously, some would say, play with the interactions of host, audience and participant, and increasingly between participants, on a world-wide stage before millions, so that they are encouraged to develop relationships, in many cases sexual, in the full glare of the TV spotlight. Here the Heart is denied the privacy and time it needs to go about the delicate and always tricky business of entering into a new relationship with another human being. Little wonder such programmes attract vast audiences of those seeking vicariously, and thus with no risk to themselves, to penetrate the subtle secrets of how the Heart works.

The pressures this era of mass communication place upon the Heart can be seen vividly, too, in the ever-increasing public acceptance of what, in previous ages, would have been considered perversions. If you work your way through late night TV channels, at some point you will come across a near-pornographic channel, accessible to the youngest child, and shocking to the eyes of those of us, like me, brought up in a more naïve world. Equally shocking can be the distortions exerted by internet chat rooms where a young girl sitting in the safety of her bedroom can indulge in sexual talk her parents drinking their coffee downstairs are unaware of. Here the line between fantasy and reality has become dangerously blurred, and the natural protection the older generation with its lifetime of experience can provide no longer exists. With the complex inventions of website and internet we have lost the age of innocence. We are all old before our time. Indeed, the young, grown blasé by exposure to this teeming world of ever more bizarre and perverse relationships, are sadly now far older and apparently more experienced than their more naïve parents. We pay for such loss of innocence in many ways, because we deny the young time to experiment in the shallows of budding relationships before they plunge into deep emotional waters, where they struggle to keep afloat.

Such a growing disregard for the sheltered havens our Heart requires in which to develop its relationships brings trouble in its wake by trivializing what should be the deepest levels of human experience. Each element experiences the stresses modern life imposes on us in differing ways. The Wood element shows its strain in the increased incidence of road and air rage, and ever-growing levels of alcohol and substance abuse, all evidence of a breakdown in its ability to control events. Fire's stress is shown by the extraordinary growth of professional helpers of all kinds, including of course acupuncturists, whose working life is devoted almost entirely to guiding their patients and clients as they attempt to sort out their relationship problems. What in the past might or might not have worked itself out through the wear and tear of a lifetime spent together, either as partners, family members or friends, without the luxury of choice, is now the subject of innumerable discussions with others outside the relationships which are causing us difficulties. Privacy is a thing of the past, as, too, is the stoicism required of us to accept our lot, however hard it may be. People of earlier ages accepted a certain level of happiness as something arising from doing one's duty. Happiness, which represents the Heart at peace, now has much more selfish aims, and ones which often conflict, since the Heart is primarily an unselfish organ.

Much of what we have discussed here places great strain upon our ability to differentiate appropriately between right and wrong for us, between what contributes to our emotional health and what distracts from it. This is properly the area of the Small Intestine. Increasingly it becomes difficult for it to assess correctly what is for our good and what is not, causing us further confusion. The morality of former ages now looks out of date, and there is little to replace it so that the moral edges become too blurred for comfort. All this puts great strain upon the Fire element whose responsibility it is to get our relationships with others right. Herein lies the Fire element's hard work, and also its great rewards if this work is done well.

CHAPTER 7

THE EARTH ELEMENT

Fire's challenge is to stay in the sunlight and to hold back the shade. And with each passing summer day its efforts grow a little more tired, until, as the daylight hours start to shorten, its domain moves inch by inch towards that of its child, Earth, the product of all its warmth, forming the hub of the circle of the elements. Bathed though we are in the remaining heat of the late summer sun, we start to feel nature turning in on itself as it foreshadows a return to the darkening days of autumn. On our journey round the elements we stand now at the crossroads, dividing north from south and east from west, drawn to Earth, the centre, as children are to their mothers, for Earth represents the mother element in all its aspects.

The two elements we have looked at so far move in one direction only, turning their faces outwards away from themselves. Wood strides forwards into the future and Fire translates this stride into a movement towards others enclosing us all in a world of relationships. Some part of Earth, like these other two elements, remains turned with its face still tilted towards the sun, but to this thrust is added a further pull towards itself.

We have seen how Wood imprints an outline upon all growing things in the shape of their buds, and Fire's warmth unfolds these into full bloom. Now here, with Earth, from all this abundant growth there comes the harvest to all these activities. The high yang activity of summer bears its fruit. The year turns slowly on its axis from yang to yin, and we move into the season we call late summer or harvest time. There is still something of the yang of high summer in the air, as the days, though gradually shortening, remain golden, and yet we start to feel the pull downwards as trees and plants tilt their burdens of fruit to the ground, yin-wards we can say.

I see how this heaviness translates itself into what is going on around me today, as I walk in the fields here in late July. Summer now has a faded look. Things are dusty and slightly stale, as though the sun has dried out all their freshness. We are barely past the summer solstice, hardly time for the dark to start encroaching on the brightness of summer's long days, and yet it is strange how soon what was once so clear and shining becomes so quickly dulled, its peak past. The leaves have a slightly shrunken look, as though frayed at their edges. There is something of a downward movement starting, as the earth draws itself inwards, saturated by the summer sun. A slight touch of heaviness in the air hints at shorter days, at an imperceptible turning of the year's tide.

This summer has been so hot and dry that it has shrivelled all the moisture from the land, bringing forward by weeks the onset of harvest. All has become yellowed by the heat of the sun, the freshness of sap within the stalks drying up to make them brittle to the touch, as though preparing themselves to be gathered in. Where there remains some green, the vegetation is still supple, as it holds on tenaciously to the last dregs of life. Here, walking in the countryside, I can hear the loud hum of the tractors as they bring in the harvest in the warm glow of a late summer evening. The corn is dry, the air heavy with dust. Even the slightest murmur of breeze seems to stir fragments of chaff in the air, as they swirl around beneath my feet. I sneeze and cough as the dry particles reach my nose. It is still very hot and yet it is not the heat of high summer. Instead I feel a loaded, heavy heat, as though the air is weighted down with it. The days are starting to draw in, minute by minute sucked in towards the dark, each lost minute of light a tiny reminder of the encroaching dark before us.

I can hear around me the steady hum and clatter of the tractors as they work upon the land, for all that abundance on earth, tree and bush must be carefully harvested before it is too late and autumn rots it underfoot. The slow pace of summer, long drawn out in the heat, quickens a little as some urgency in the air makes us aware that we must rouse ourselves from our langour and fight against a tide of warm inertia to bring in what we need if we are not to pass empty-handed into autumn, our larders bare.

Each fruit contains within it all that bud and blossom together have created, drawn into a concentrated kernel of nourishment. Apple, nut and tomato, the blackberry and the rosehip, all are products of the abundance that has gone before, condensed down into forms small enough to provide nourishment for living things. The expansion of Wood and Fire is now sucked inwards to form the products of Earth's work, small parcels of food, ready to be released when they are ripe. Out of the earth has grown the bud to become the tree, to become the fruit, now ripe and full, hanging on its branches. We need only stand below those heavily laden trees for food to fall down into our opened mouths. And out here in nature I can see why the Earth part of us is our home, providing the food that we eat and the resting-place beneath our feet, our mother element, strongly associated with how we relate to our birth mother.

But it does not only represent the fruits which it offers us as sustenance. It is also the ground upon which these fruits are grown. It is below the highest mountain and the deepest cavern. It is a desert, a rocky place, a deep cold ravine. It can be shifting sands, or the hard rock upon which the great oceans rest. Its great belly can swell with trees, heave with mountains, suck itself into the deepest valleys, or lie flattened over the plains. Upon its body grows everything we need to support life.

Fire lives its life openly and centre-stage. Its learning is done in the public eye, and its mistakes and successes are there for all to see. It signals its presence from afar, for it is always visible, blazing forth even in the darkness of the night. As it announces whatever it does to all around, there, deep down below its feet and tucked firmly out of sight, lies hidden its sister element, risking much less, and wiser in keeping its counsel. Like some mother cat watching her kittens playing over her, Earth allows us to make sport upon her. She is an indulgent mother, always there whatever we do to her, as all mothers should be. She moves slowly, for she carries the whole world upon her back. Her function is to establish and consolidate, not to do, but to be. Life seeps into Earth. It waits to be done unto, a ground upon which others sow and reap.

Earth underlies everything, and is there where everything happens, for everything that happens has to happen upon its face. It has no need to move outwards to find things, as Fire does. Things find their way home to it. Gravity draws us back firmly to its bosom, however much we may long to be free to fly away. People scurry along and scratch its surface, busily running their little lives, whilst below mile upon mile of impenetrable Earth rests upon itself, steady, deep, unmoving, our still firm centre.

But what if the pressures of life upon it prevent it from maintaining its stability and threaten its calm surface? Ripples of unrest can run through rock, for whole cities, built upon its solid foundations, can be reduced to rubble by the merest twinge shaking Earth's body. Earthquakes can destroy in moments what it has taken us centuries to build. Every now and again, as a reminder of Earth's shadow-side, its belly, belching smoke and molten rock, is rent apart to reveal the very torments of hell lying beneath our pleasant meadows, gentle streams and waving corn. Even the great masses of solid rock below our feet can offer us no protection. Earth tucks itself deeply away within itself in an attempt to avoid acknowledging its own insecurity, but its bed heaves and shakes beneath it.

Where Fire will signal its distresses to all, Earth turns back into itself and buries deep to hide its pain. It hides from itself within itself. This can be its natural defence, or its shadow side. If the pressures of life become too great, it will just disappear inside itself. In that sense, despite its great solidity and sheer presence, it is an elusive element, for we do not know where it is. All but the tiny part of it visible on the surface always remains hidden. When life disturbs it, it creeps down and becomes almost invisible. It has so much of itself to hide within. This is a necessary defence, much as Fire, more visible, hides behind its smiles. Earth, under attack, must know how to retreat into itself, but when out of control its natural desire to remain hidden becomes too effective a cover, enabling it to disappear within itself and never find itself again. Since it is everywhere, it is so easy for it to merge undifferentiated into the whole, its sense of identity becoming lost in those depths.

Stability, strength, duration, support, nourishment and the calmness of just being, these are Earth's great blessings. They are shadowed by impermanence, instability and the terror of not being. If the very rocks beneath our feet can be split asunder by the merest rumble within Earth's flank, then there is nothing stable under the sun to which we can cling. We perch insecurely where we imagined ourselves to be safely anchored. Earth teaches us that we must learn to rely for support on nobody but ourselves.

The pull of Earth

The tug to itself which we experience as one of Earth's qualities is that which differentiates Earth most strongly from Fire, the two elements most closely associated with the people who surround them. The movement of Fire is a form of stretching out towards others. Here, with Earth, that movement is in the opposite direction, where the love once offered us by Fire is now demanded back by Earth.

There is always about Earth a drawing quality, as of something pulling us towards its centre, a quality we recognize physically as the pull of gravity upon us, drawing us back to the earth beneath our feet. Gravity is the physical web the universe weaves around us and from which we can only momentarily escape by those acts of daring, our flights through space, tiny challenges we throw at the cosmos in defiance of the tight grip with which it holds us girdled to the earth. It creates so strong a pull that not even the greatest athlete can withstand it for longer than the few seconds it takes the high-jumper to jump a bare few feet from the ground before being dragged back, or the slightly longer time it takes a pole-vaulter, aided by his pole, to propel himself a few, so very few, more feet into the sky. And we know how much power is needed to drag an aeroplane into the sky and keep it up there, and even more to propel a rocket beyond gravity's pull.

And we experience Earth's pull all the time, and yet usually remain completely unaware of it, unless, as happened to me recently, something makes us conscious of it. I was lying in my bath, lazily waiting for the water to drain away before climbing out, and as it did so I slowly felt my skin being sucked earthwards by so strong a force that I felt I was experiencing something of the suction I have seen reflected on astronauts' faces as their rocket leaves the earth's atmosphere. It may seem an exaggerated comparison, that of an astronaut in outer space with me in my bath, and yet so strong was my body's reaction to regaining its sensation of weight that the example is no idle one. If you experience this for yourself it will give you some inkling of the centrifugal force to which the Earth element is always subject. And this pull is echoed in all it does. It draws all towards it, as the hub of a wheel draws to itself the axles' power to make the wheel go round.

In much earlier times, before the chart of the five element circle moved it to the outer periphery, the Earth element was sited at the centre, with the other elements circling round it as its spokes. In many ways this represents a truer picture of its pivotal role, an axis, a form of crossroads, through which all things pass on their way outwards to the other elements. And just as a hub turns more slowly than the spokes rotating by its power, so Earth people have something of a similar slowness as they wait to process the activities of others, a form of passivity no Wood or Fire person has, for even when these two elements are out of balance something of that outward-turning movement remains in them, however hidden, to be expressed in the smiles of Fire or the restlessness of Wood.

A sensation of lurking heaviness accompanies Earth people wherever they move (and I suspect perhaps few of them would opt to be high-jumpers!), and is one of the reasons why it is often Earth people who find flying difficult, for here, in leaving the ground, they are forcing their bodies away from that safe attachment to the earth beneath their feet which they crave, the act of leaving the ground representing for some an extreme disconnection, as though they are severing the umbilical cord attaching them to the earth. And to some extent this is true for all of us, however we may disguise it, as we experience a moment of brief terror as we soar upwards. I am always fascinated by the complete silence which falls upon an aeroplane filled with hardened travellers as it takes off and again as it lands, as though, for those few moments, we are all suddenly reminded of our audacity in thus defying nature's pull.

Earth's need must necessarily be first to itself, for no plant can grow fruit if it is not properly nourished, and this gives it the two-way movement so characteristic of its position as the pivot of the elements. It takes and then gives, giving only when what it has taken has nourished it sufficiently. And this it does not only in terms of the physical food we need to nourish ourselves with, but also of our thoughts and feelings. For the activity of processing, the churning over of things to extract their fruit, like a combine harvester extracting grain from corn stalks, is one of the gifts Earth brings to all its activities, extending to the fruits of our inner world. These, too, it processes, being the most thoughtful of all elements in its attempts to extract sustenance and understanding from what it draws deep within it. It can ponder long before it digests a thought, only extracting from it a meaning, a fruit, after much work is done. Other elements will take advantage of its efforts to help them speed their own thoughts, none more so than its child, the Metal element, which builds upon Earth's processing to form conclusions with a speed and acuteness which Earth can only dream of. But then Metal's task, as we shall see, is quite other.

An element in distress will look outside itself for what it is unable to provide for itself, those very gifts which are its unique inheritance turning into burdens too heavy to bear. They become a focal point for dissatisfaction, for each guardian is aware of its own failure to offer what it should, chiding itself constantly for its own lack of generosity. A gauge of an element's importance to each of us are those areas where we show the greatest unease, for they are pointers to something we are trying desperately to reach, but which eludes our grasp. Just as Wood, out of balance, makes its way towards an existence structured and planned by others, and Fire attempts to spread love and warmth where none is wanted, Earth demands the nourishment from all around that it should itself be providing. When out of balance, Earth can ache with the pain of hunger, and, like some parched and arid desert, can give nothing of itself when it has nothing left to give. Denied its own nourishment, it must hold to itself all that it can so generously bestow, else it will starve, and thus if it is troubled, it has to become selfish. Taking what it should be giving, it stands hungry before its own empty larder, demanding of others that they replenish it.

Whenever we are distressed, we hoard greedily to ourselves the gifts we should be sharing, for in that distress we have no way of knowing whether, in giving, we may not be emptying ourselves of all that we have. Each element has its own particular neediness, that of Wood, for the whole world to be ordered to its liking, that of Fire, for the whole world to accept its love, and now that of Earth, for the whole world to feed it, for deep within Earth, where Fire aches with endless love, lies the ghost of a starving child.

Our relationship to food is dictated to a large extent by the degree of nurturing we receive from our mother. It is further shaped by the way in which this nurturing, both physical and emotional, is given us. A meal turned out on to a cold plate from a tin will not nourish any of us, least of all a baby with its subtle senses, as much as a lovingly prepared meal which starts to stimulate our taste buds as it is cooked, and is presented as part of the communal activity of a shared meal taken at leisure around a table. That table, surrounded by family members and friends, is a symbol of the Earth element's role at the centre. Such an image should be before us when we think of this element, replete and satisfied, deeply nourished and thus now, at last, able to nourish others.

The two officials which carry out Earth's functions within us are the Stomach and the Spleen. The Stomach processes all the activities of body and soul, and the Spleen transports the results of these activities throughout body and soul. The Stomach can be regarded as a kind of cement mixer, churning things over that come to it, breaking them down into ever smaller parts and then passing them on to the Spleen to carry along like some endless conveyor belt. And, here, too, in their positioning on our bodies we see demonstrated the Earth element's slightly curious position at our centre, for these two officials, the one yang, the other yin, are the only two which lie close to one another on the surface of the body as they pass over those important areas, the chest and abdomen, only branching slightly to inner and outer sides of the body as they reach the thigh and leg. All other yin/yang pairings of officials follow different courses along the body, either on the back (yang) and front (yin), or on the outside areas of the body (yang) as opposed to the inner and central (yin). With this element, by contrast, we see the Stomach take its place firmly next to its yin official, the Spleen, and, yang though it is, it runs over the most yin aspect of all, our nipple, as though staking a claim to unite yin and yang in this way.

Earth is the great container, bearing within it the weight of the whole world. Earth's great learning is to break loose from itself to stand alone. Its challenge is to free itself from its own company. Its fear is that it might never know what life is, eternally a dead planet, unquickened. It fears that it may never be brought to life. Fire's fear is that it might never know what love is, its heart eternally cold. It fears it may never be brought to love. Wood's fear is that it will be denied growth, a bud forever closed. It fears it may never be allowed to unfold.

Earth is the hearth in which Fire burns upon the kindling Wood provides.

Princess Diana

The Earth element imprints itself upon us in a yellow colour which in balance is like that of ripe golden corn, its smell is sweet, and the sound of its voice has a lilt to it, we call by the name of singing. We call its emotion, among other things, sympathy, the ability to feel not so much for somebody else, which is the meaning we usually give this word in English, but with somebody, as in the original Greek word. It can also be called pensiveness, expressing that aspect of its character concerned with the processing of thought. We have seen that life can be said to seep into Earth. It is not an activator, as are Wood or Fire. It works upon the materials which it is given, receiving and transforming them within us, as thought, feeling or food, into a form we can digest. If we imagine the earth beneath our feet awaiting the rain to fall to make it fertile, or the seed within it to burst into life, we have an image before us of the way in which Earth takes unto itself the emotions others are feeling and then makes them its own. This taking in and processing activity represents what we call the emotion sympathy in its widest sense.

If we feel what a friend is feeling, we can convey this feeling to her by our understanding, and she will regard this understanding as an expression of sympathy. If I am in distress, somebody showing me that they understand how I feel will be viewed as a sympathetic person. They are showing that they understand what I am going through, and in so doing they are offering me solace. I feel better for this comfort, whether it is wordless or not, my burden for a moment lessened as I feel it shared by another. This is an example of how we expect this emotion to show itself in Earth people in balance. They are able to absorb into themselves my feelings of distress and transform them inside themselves into some verbal or physical expression of sympathetic understanding (through caring eyes, a warm word or a touch, for example), by which I recognize the reciprocation of my feelings. This ability to comfort, much as a mother is asked to comfort a child, is a gift the Earth element within all of us can bestow.

But how comforting the level of empathy is that Earth can show will depend on various factors. All dominant characteristics which the guardian element bestows upon us are placed under constant strain as our element attempts to keep itself on track. Wood may respond inappropriately to others' anger, Fire to others' joy or inability to show joy. Earth can respond inappropriately to the demands of others for sympathy and understanding. This element, which on the face of it should appear to be the kindest of all, the mother element there to feed us all, may therefore become excessively unmotherly when itself in need. And then its capacity for sympathy can turn to a hardness, a denial of sympathy, if too much is asked of it, so that what in balance is the most understanding of elements can become instead the hardest of all when out of balance, denying others the right to be offered the understanding and nourishment it feels it is itself denied. It may also reveal its imbalance by exaggerating its concern. Bland expressions, such as 'Oh, you poor thing', or 'How terrible', uttered without feeling, then become a way of distancing themselves from the problems of others which drain them with their demands. Here the giving and taking which is Earth's nature sends out confusing signals as the expected appropriate emotional response of sympathy is withheld. Earth people will always have this twofold quality. In their giving they will always retain a part that seeks to take, and in their taking they will always in part be giving.

And perhaps there is no better example of seeing this demonstrated than in that most famous of all Earth people, Princess Diana, in whom an extreme need to give was so counterbalanced by an extreme need to take that some people regarded her as totally selfish, whilst to others she was supremely unselfish. And indeed she could be said to have been both at the same time. This is made clear in that famous television interview in which she invited the whole world to bear witness to her need for sympathy, whilst at the same time she was occupied in helping starving children and Aids victims, and fighting, undoubtedly absolutely with genuine conviction, for the banning of landmines. There can be no more vivid an illustration of these two often conflicting sides of the Earth element.

And her pleading voice, with the lullaby lilt all Earth people have, demanded of the millions of us who watched her that we look after her and mother her like some child, as she gratefully received our outpourings of sympathy. And when she died, the grief of those to whom she had in turn offered sympathy, the maimed and the marginalized, was a genuine reflection of her capacity to offer others what she craved for herself. She was able to feed them as she demanded in turn to be fed by them. And her needs were extreme, because her life was lived in the harshness of the public gaze as the most famous woman on the planet, and thus she demanded extreme satisfactions, to the extent that the attentions of photographers who pursued her were so necessary to her that she deliberately called them to her to witness her private moments.

And as witnesses we were indeed confused, and often exasperated, by her conflicting needs, which expressed themselves, appropriately for the Earth element, amongst other things in her eating disorders. Here Earth's organ, the Stomach, proves unable to feed itself properly, one minute gorging itself, the next emptying itself. If we recall that she lost her mother when she was a young girl, it may well be that she never fully recovered from the absence of that mothering all of us need before we can in turn nourish ourselves and others properly.

She was said to be a devoted mother (unselfishly giving), but was quite happy to allow her children to witness her attack upon their father in front of an audience of millions (selfishly taking). Nothing could satisfy her, not even the adulation of these millions. You can have no greater example of the Earth element standing before its own empty larder. Here, visibly, we can see the ghost of that starving child, abandoned in childhood by her mother and seeking always, it seemed, for comfort and nourishment from all around her throughout a short and tragic life.

To what we have learnt about Earth I will add a further example from my own practice to illustrate some of its qualities in greater detail. I have chosen a patient of mine, Andy, who has been coming to me for more than ten years. He originally sought help because he felt that his life had reached some kind of impasse. He is in his 50s, a business man with a chain of shops. He sees his treatments as a way of ensuring that he remains in balance, and appreciates the support and understanding I give him which is what his element needs. When he came this week he lay down on the treatment couch with a sigh, tucked himself cosily under the blanket and launched into a long account of what had gone on since last I saw him.

He always sets his own agenda. There are certain things he has come to tell me about and he has to tell them in a certain order and in a certain way. He is disconcerted if I interrupt him, as though I am disturbing the train of his thought and speech. Anything I interject which halts this flow appears to disrupt a thought process which has its own cadences, and I must take care not to break this cycle. My contributions are welcome, but only if these do not impede the flow of what he is saying. Any clumsy interruption on my part is as though I have knocked the cement mixer so that its flow falters. The words dry up on his lips, a puzzled look will appear on his face, as though he finds it difficult to re-align his thoughts again, and I have to wait until he has got his thought processes re-started before he can go on talking. When interrupted in this way, he carries on at exactly the same point in his story at which I have broken in upon him, almost as though he has not heard my interruption.

He needs to draw me into his world, swallow me with every mouthful as it were. I am asked to be part of the processing of what he does, my input only essential in that I must not impede this churning over of thought in any way. Thus any interruption to the wheels of thought turning round in his mind are seen as jarring, and will often be ignored as though they have not even been heard, so intent is he upon this inward-turning movement of cogitation. Possibly the nod of a head or a murmur to show that I have heard and understood is more essential than I realize, for this indicates to him that I am taking in what he is telling me, and the taking in of things is what is so important of Earth. A participating audience may indeed be needed as a sign of that participation, as though I am like some ingredient thrown with all those other thoughts and impressions into Earth's mouth, like water into a concrete mixer, or oil into the mechanism which turns it round.

This sense of circular thought is very characteristic of the Earth element. We have seen that Earth's function is to process what comes to it until it has changed it into a form it can digest. This churning process transforms the original ingredients into something new, smoother, more malleable. This is similar to our chewing our food over before swallowing it to create the nutrients by which we survive. The Earth carries on this continuous processing work, much as a mother transforms the food and water she ingests into the milk which will feed her baby. As Andy lies there telling me what he has come to tell me about, the raw ingredients of his thoughts are already in him when he arrives, and I can see his mind churning these thoughts over to produce speech as he talks. He is looking in towards himself, as befits that inward-turning movement of Earth.

And, too, Earth, being the centre, needs others around it whatever it does, disliking working in isolation for too long. The thought processing which is one of its tasks needs the kind of grist to the mill provided by others' thoughts and interactions, a constant input from outside necessary for assimilation to take place. It is difficult to chew with an empty mouth, or indeed on an empty stomach, the saliva soon drying up if no other nutrients are introduced. And this is an apt metaphor for the kind of dry and painful processing Earth people can engage in. It also illustrates something essential to Earth, the fact that this most potentially fertile of all elements is basically sterile until other elements plant their seeds in it, provide it with air and water and ripen it to maturity. This explains the feelings of emptiness all Earth people can experience at intervals, as though starved of all nourishment.

With Andy, then, I feel that my function is to nourish him with my offerings of thoughts and above all my understanding, all a form of input demanded of me to feed what can seem like an endless cycle of need. But I am not required to intercede in the actual processing itself, which Earth regards as its task to perform unaided. He is also much occupied with himself, the centre of his universe formed by the 'I' of his existence. However devoted a husband and father he is, and he is undoubtedly that, the centre of gravity around which his family revolves is his own sense of himself. Once this sense of the importance of his own personal identity is lost, which happens when he is out of balance, Earth's innate selfishness, its over-dependence on self as the pivot of its existence, reasserts itself to the point where it is unable to take account of others' needs. Andy showed this side of himself this week, for he was restless and ill at ease, trying to work out a new direction to his life now that his family is moving away. He feels that its centre is slowly shifting away from him, and this feels threatening to one for whom this pivotal position in the family, as in life in general, is all important. It is as though the wheel of which he forms the hub has been moved slightly out of alignment, disturbing the pattern of his life.

Since coming for treatment, the sensory signals he used to send out have changed. The dirty yellow colour he showed initially has changed to the clear golden glow which we recognize as that of Earth in balance. His smell has changed from a slightly cloying smell to a pleasant sweet smell we call fragrant. And his emotion which initially was something akin to an inability to show any sympathy at all, has softened to allow him to express his natural ability to empathize with others more easily. The lilting sound to his voice has dropped its exaggerated overtones, and has become softer and less demanding of its listeners.

The feeling I experience as Andy's practitioner is of being pulled to the centre of a circular movement. With James, my Wood patient, I am confronted, engaged directly, not necessarily for what I offer in my own right so much as a sparring partner, somebody against whom he can find his own boundaries, as though he will need eventually to push past me to get to his goal. With Rebecca, my Fire patient, I am face to face, but I feel I am of personal interest to her and have in that sense entered into a relationship with her, where in James' case I feel who I am is not as important as what I can offer him. These are essential characteristics of the three elements we have looked at so far which help us to pinpoint some of those subtle differences which distinguish each of their manifestations.

And if my mother, Princess Diana or Billy Connolly had all been my patients, they would have demanded different things from me as their practitioner, their demands reflecting their different elements. My mother would have wanted a brisk, cheerful professionalism, yielding quick results, Diana my close and undivided attention to every aspect of her life and the time to listen to her, and Billy Connolly would try to shrug off his problems by somehow wanting me to laugh at them with him. If I had offered to Princess Diana what Billy Connolly would have been comfortable with, she would have felt disappointed because I was not letting her speak her thoughts out. In turn, if I gave Billy Connolly the sympathetic attention with which I would listen to Princess Diana, he would have found this distasteful. My mother, though liking a bit of sympathy, too, was also capable of laughing at herself, but both of these only up to a point. Both the sympathy and the ability to find things ridiculous were peripheral to her need for quick results.

The elements in embryo

It is interesting at this stage to extend our understanding of the Earth element by looking at another of its most fundamental manifestations in each of our lives, one which we have to draw on first in the womb and then increasingly less often in infancy and childhood, that of the nurturing role our mother plays in our physical development. For it is through the initial work of our mother's officials that our own gradually learn to assume the responsibilities which will become totally theirs as we take on an independent existence.

Embedded as we are within our mother from the time of conception to the time of our birth, each of our cells remains alive only through what she provides us with. It is her Lung which draws in air for us to survive, her Heart which first supplies the beat and the blood flow which eventually creates our own heart and circulatory system, her Stomach and other officials which process the food she eats and breaks it down into nutrients sufficiently small to pass through the placenta into our own bodies, her Large Intestine which gets rid of our baby waste. To and fro through the placental fluid her own officials feed her growing baby's developing officials with what they need. And the process is not merely at the physical level. Each of these officials, as we have seen, has an emotional sphere specific to it. And these must develop well before birth, in tandem with the physical development of our organs.

Thus, at the same time as the tiny embryo starts to process food as its physical stomach develops, it also starts to think and process these thoughts, and gradually to develop the capacity to think of others which will eventually enable it to offer them sympathy. It will take time for it to develop the capacity to transform these thoughts into words, but well before this we can see how carefully a tiny baby studies it surroundings as it tries to absorb all the many happenings in this vibrant new world into which it has emerged. And each official is similarly stimulated to develop its particular function, at both a physical and emotional level, these two processes moving forward in parallel. This work will start first in the womb, which is where our connection to the Earth element in its nurturing capacity is the strongest, but continues well into childhood and then adulthood, and indeed may never be said to cease, so strong is the band tying us through our umbilical cord to our mother and the Earth element which she represents.

From our knowledge of physiology, we know that different organs develop at different times within the embryo. So, too, do these organs' emotional companions, some requiring longer, much longer to develop than their physical counterparts. The long maturation process of the human being, who moves into adulthood only in late teens (if then, or if ever!), is mirrored by the gradual development of a maturing emotional structure in which the officials slowly learn to balance their emotional needs as appropriately as possible. We could be said to be fortunate in having at our sides what we would hope would be the wise companionship of older family members to guide us through the emotional minefields which represent a young person's induction into adult life. We know that, all too often, this is sadly not what happens, and that this guidance may fall far short of what is needed, but the ideal situation would reflect the kind of nurturing and protecting of its young we see adult animals do so unselfishly in all the nature programmes on TV which fascinate so many of us, perhaps because among other things they recall for us a paradise of parental care often only too far removed from that we receive in this modern world.

Vestiges of the mature functions of each element are present in the baby, as seeds of their final, mature growth. Just as a mother filters the food for her baby through herself to make it digestible for its embryonic stomach, first in the womb and then from some months after birth in her milk, so all the experiences a baby undergoes are filtered in some way through its parents and immediate surroundings as it lies helpless in its cot. Later its mother will mash its food with a fork or give it ready-prepared food from a jar, much like a mother bird does for its chick, in a slightly different way, but for exactly the same reasons. It takes at least 4–5 months before the child is able to take on solids of any kind, and it will continue to drink milk in one form or another as its staple food well into its first few years. Parents will also act as processors and interpreters of those other things, apart from food, which the baby will be expected to absorb from its environment.

It will be helpful to approach an understanding of this development from the perspective of the human baby who emerges into life only half-formed, and has to learn gradually to assume control of its body and its environment, until with time it is able to survive independently without outside help. This gradual learning process is guided by the energies of the different elements, as they bring to maturity the organs and functions over which they have control.

I will use the Fire element to illustrate how delicate are the processes by which our maturing officials learn to assume their functions, and how prey they are to attack. The Heart is the first official to develop as an organ, but its emergence depends upon the earlier development of two of its protector officials, the Three Heater, the body's thermostat, and the Heart Protector, which controls our blood circulation. These two functions are the earliest to emerge as our growing cells divide and have the widest remit of all the officials, underpinning the work of all the others. It is by their actions that the Heart can unfold within the embryo. Like tiny buds opening up and fanning out to bring life to one cell after another, these two officials perfuse the developing embryo with sufficient blood and heat to allow the Heart to form, before it in turn starts to pump forth the blood to create and keep alive organ after organ. Each organ can be seen as another bud slowly unfolding within us, linked each to the next like buds on a twig, their life-giving sap our blood, each bursting slowly open to form the mature organs with their complex interacting functions, all of which are essential to our growth.

Vulnerable as we are to outside pressures for so many more years than our animal counterparts, we are all too exposed to the effects of any imbalances in those surrounding us with what we hope is love and protection. I often think it is surprising that any of us moves towards maturity in the balanced state some of us, at least, do, so overwhelming is the pressure upon us exerted by a life lived in this overcrowded planet of ours, teeming with millions of others determined to fight for their own small space to survive. Our officials, requiring many years to assume full responsibility and working against such a confused background, are often given insufficient support during this long process to develop in a balanced way, and here none are more vulnerable than the Fire officials, with the Heart, our most important organ, in their midst.

But when we are newborn, these functions, like everything else about us, will still be at the very earliest stages of their development, and have to be nurtured with help from our parents. How successfully the child starts to take over this role itself will depend upon how well the parents upon whom it relies for protection are able to fulfil this protective role. For example, it will be to a parent that a baby looks for help in judging whether a situation or person is safe or dangerous, precisely the function the Heart's protective mechanisms perform. And without an adult's help a baby cannot put on the outer coverings it needs to survive even on the mildest summer's day, or take them off again if it gets too hot, and it takes quite a few years before it can adjust its clothing appropriately by itself. In the early days of a baby's life, parents and close family therefore act at one level as its Heart Protector, its Small Intestine and its Three Heater officials, forming a first line of defence for the baby's vulnerable Heart. The Fire element's functions which govern the Heart and its protector meridians will be present in a baby, but in immature form, awaiting the instructions life provides to encourage them to develop to their full.

The Wood officials, too, can provide a further example of the gradual development of their role on our journey from embryo to full adult. We know that they control the articulation of all the actions of body and soul, and are concerned with every aspect of planning and decision-making. If we look at a baby emerging into the world at birth, very little about its movements is structured or co-ordinated. Among the numerous things it cannot yet do is focus its eyes, control its limbs or formulate the differentiated sounds we recognize as speech. Compare this with yourself as you read this now. you will be holding this book in your hands, your eyes will be scanning the words, your brain will be interpreting the meaning of the symbols on the page, you will be telling your fingers to turn to the next page when it is time to do so, and you are at the same time holding yourself upright in your chair. If somebody calls out to you, you will lift your head to see who it is and reply in words we can all understand.

Perhaps, as we saw with the decision to make a cup of tea in Chapter 5, you tire of reading and decide to take a break, giving all the necessary instructions to your mind and body to get up from your chair and get some refreshment. All of these actions will probably be below the conscious level, so integrated has the act of reading and the act of taking a break become into our lives, but watch a little child trying to pronounce its first words or take its first steps, and you will see how intricate are the processes involved and how complex is the learning required to achieve such simple actions.

The development towards maturity involves us moving from total dependency upon our mother to emergence as a semi-independent being at birth and on towards total independence. In acupuncture terms this movement is seen as the work of the elements as their different officials gradually form organs and body parts, and encourage these one by one to assume their own functions, with the elements within the mother gradually teaching the elements within the child the tasks necessary for the child to survive.

CHAPTER 8

The Metal Element

And it is a truism, often repeated, to say that we somehow never really escape from our mothers, for we continue to rely for survival on the food which initially they alone could provide us with, demanding it now from the earth beneath our feet. Nor, in a completely different way, can we escape our fathers, for we will see as we now move on to the Metal element that it is this element which provides us throughout our life with that most precious and rarefied gift, the air we breathe, and complements the Earth element by representing the father's role in the family of elements. And to this element we now turn, as we reach autumn, and ask ourselves what this season brings to the cycle of life which will help us understand Earth's offspring, the Metal element.

Once the harvest has been gathered, what then? What of the fruit of the fruit? If all is not to go to waste, then some further product must emerge from the activities of the three elements that have gone before, else all their work will become meaningless. As the days shorten further, we start to move from the centre outwards, away from the light towards which Wood and Fire move us, back towards the dark. The year closes in further as the days shorten, grow darker, and autumn starts to spread itself upon the land. This is a season of passing glory, echoing the transience of life and our own troubled uncertainties in the face of this unalterable fact. It is the most vivid of all seasons, bringing its splendour to bear upon all things as it flares up briefly before fading to nothing. Our mood becomes more sombre as we view the death of the year and with it our own death. Dust to dust and ashes to ashes.

In Metal we come face to face with ourselves, and must decide whether we like what we see.

I am walking today amongst the detritus of the year, my feet at each step shuffling aside great compost heaps of dead or dying leaves, some to my surprise still clinging on tenaciously to the last drops of life. Squirrels scamper around me, scratching at the soil to draw some last kernel of nourishment from the husks of chestnuts and other fruit lying buried underfoot. A strong smell of decay rises up as I push the leaves aside, a sharp reminder of Metal's smell upon the human body, reflecting the fermenting activity our bodies have to undergo before we separate the useful from the useless and discard the waste. All Earth's products which have not been eaten or stored away are fermenting below my feet, allowing for yet another, more rarefied harvest. This is not the gross matter which feeds our stomachs, but the precious essences extracted from it, both material and spiritual, which make meaningful all that has gone before. Physically, the earth yields from this fermentation the trace elements without which nothing can grow or thrive. The yield at a deeper level is a sense of our achievements and with them some pride in what we have done.

This is truly the fall of the year, a time when all nature's energy is drawn down into the ground. Here the yin energies of the dark overcome the last of the year's yang energy, and we reach the end of that visible activity started with Wood. We enter a melancholy season where all the work of the other seasons could seem to have been as nought, a futile attempt to stave off death. Metal brings about a form of closure, as one cycle comes to an end, and another lies in waiting hidden from sight deep in winter.

The air feels lifeless, weighed down. Some trees look dead already, their branches bare of all but a few discoloured and limp leaves. The crackle of the dead leaves underfoot, the crunch of their dryness, further accentuates the increasing withdrawal of life around me. Dead leaves take up so little space on the earth. They can be crushed to dust between my fingers. No longer glorious with life, they appear to have used up whatever vitality was left in them which has leached out into the soil beneath. The feeling in the air is so unlike the expectancy of spring, for it foreshadows a preparation for the rites of death and the closure of the year. People walk looking down, as though in mourning, as they feel the hush of the land.

The afternoon light lies over all things, silent and still, heralding the approach of night. A little sunlight still glimmers through the thinning trees, making the dark branches stand out more clearly. The few remaining yellow leaves appear more yellow, almost translucent in this penetrating low light. In the late afternoon splendour, the silver birch stands as though illuminated, its delicate leaves hanging suspended like lace, moving slightly as though lifted by some unseen current of air. The late berries lie crushed red against the rocks. All is light, space and colour, for I am surrounded by colour here in the hills, immersed in it, as though enfolded in yellows, oranges, reds and dark browns, all glorious against a bright blue autumn sky. Everything is stark and clear. Enough leaves have fallen to allow the outlines of the branches to appear thinly through the yellowing background, giving a sharper focus to what I see. The lines nature is drawing are clearer now than in summer, when the warm sunlight drew all things out to their fullest, filling the skyline with an abundance of growth. Here in the creeping barrenness of autumn all things start to separate out again, making distinct each branch and twig.

I am standing looking at a spread of bright red lichen at my feet, its colour awesome in its splendour. Death is in the air and yet here is a defiant outburst of blood-red life. A small shoot growing out of the ground displays a similar declaration of the durability of life in the face of its inevitable extinction, glowing orange in all its small leaves. Thus does Metal make meaningful what can be seen as the meaninglessness of each tiny span of life. Here, with the last breath of autumn, is a celebration of life at its most awe-inspiring, its most triumphant. The autumn landscape, alight with the most ardent of colours, has about it something more of bravery and death-defying splendour than do the more strident expressions of life which spring and summer with all their vigour show me. I draw in my breath with a wonder here that no earlier flourishes of the landscape have given me, awed by the late-flowering expression of life in the face of imminent extinction. This vehement affirmation of our continuing existence despite all that tells me that life must end inspires me, each autumn a tiny foreshadowing of our eventual death.

I can feel winter starting to close in. The air is slightly fresher against my cheeks and I see slight tremors of mist rising in front of me as my warm breath meets the cooling air. Even the ferns seem to have shrunk into themselves a little more, their filaments rusty and crinkled. The fir trees alone retain an abundance of living green, evidence of life still on display despite the drawing in of light, each tree a signal of permanence against the transient background of dying leaves. They are the only truly dark objects remaining as I look around, except for the sharp outlines of trunks and branches and the deep shadows thrown by the lowering sun. In autumn we see the essence of things starkly revealed in the final fling of the year's glory.

There is a hint of stillness which presages the deep quiescence of winter. This is no active season. It does not do, but takes in, as though drawing in the final breaths of the year, accepting now that all that has been is past and must be done with, disposed of in some way, made relevant or discarded as useless, a thing of no further value except for what it has already yielded. And how are we to judge such value? That is indeed Metal's dilemma.

Metal rules over the widest domain of all the elements, extending from the Lungs as our organ of intake to the Large Intestine, our principal organ of excretion. It connects us through our breath to the vast breath of the universe rhythmically breathing in and out beyond us. And this awareness of all that lies beyond itself draws Metal's attention away from the small considerations of our everyday life up towards those things which soar eternally beyond life and death. Metal forms our bridge to the great worlds beyond. And its task is to translate all that happens within the tiny, apparently insignificant span of each of our lives into something of meaning within the greater context of all that exists.

Metal waits until the bustle of spring and summer is past before setting to work to pare away all that is insignificant, retaining only that which it considers worth keeping if the future is to gain any value from its past. If life is to be worth anything, it is Metal that assesses what that worth could be. Where Fire weighs all things upon the scales of love, Metal weighs them upon the scales of their value. Its task is to ensure that the great cycle of activity starting with Wood does not fade away into insignificance.

Metal represents not only the air we breathe, but also that essence which nature passes on to feed the renewal of life each year. Not all withers away to nothing in autumn. The dead leaves, broken down by the forces of rain and wind, release into the ground trace elements which nourish the ground in which the future seed will grow. The quality of what has been deposited in the soil in autumn will determine the strength of next year's growth. Without air, nothing can live, and without trace elements the soil cannot nurture the rebirth of life. Without Metal's quality, the work of all the other elements would be as nothing, valueless. So strong is Metal's determination to deal only with what is valuable and pure, that it will set itself and others the highest standards, often finding it difficult itself to live up to them. Metal is a perfectionist, being unable to finish a thing until it is exactly as it wants it. It has difficulty in accepting that it has done the best it can, because that best is never enough. And having always some lingering suspicion that it could have done better, it can be reluctant to let things go.

In its search for what lies beyond itself, Metal always feels there is something out there which it must strive to reach. In balance, it will experience this as something further on, beyond it, a goal to be achieved. Out of balance, it will experience this as something further back which has eluded it, an opportunity missed, a cause for regret. Metal is the element that most sighs for what might have been and now can never be. Once its energy becomes unbalanced, this sense of past failure can become so crippling that a person lives only in the past, looking back with longing eyes to a time when things might have been different. And this yearning for some past time which never was can cut Metal people off from the present, making them feel as though they are no longer connected to things. Life can then seem empty and meaningless, its purpose no longer clear.

And there is a sadness deep within Metal, for this seeker after the perfect knows that, search as it will, it can never find the perfect thing for which it is looking. It weeps for all our imperfections. It weeps because it knows that at the heart of Wood's bud of hope lies nestling death, life's eternal shadow. Thus grief is Metal's emotion. Its colour is white, the colour of the shroud, its smell is that of autumn leaves trodden underfoot, and its voice weeps for the passing of all things.

Lung, Metal's yin official, is, with Stomach, our main organ of intake. Physically, it inhales air. At the deeper level within us it is there to absorb all those things which come to us from outside, others' thoughts and ideas, those impressions of what is around us which we need to take in and make our own. As it does with the air we breathe, the things which impinge upon us from the world outside cannot be received by us without Lung's filter, that first stage on the process of transformation from without to within. It is therefore quite clear why the Chinese called the skin, also under this official's protection, our third lung, its pores each a tiny receptor turned towards the outside world, breathing in air and passing the product of each of these in-breaths on to the blood.

To allow us room constantly to take new things in, some of what we take in has to be released, either in the form of waste products, the waste material of all those acts of transformation we undergo within ourselves, or of releasing from ourselves whatever we wish to pass on to the world outside. This is the Large Intestine's function, as it continues the process of purification which the Lung has started. We should breathe in only clean, fresh air, and the Lung uses little filters in our nose to sift through each breath of air and ensure it will not harm us. The Large Intestine helps in this cleansing process by expelling polluted air by making us cough, for here Chinese medicine has a much wider grasp of this organ of elimination, seeing it as its most important task to expel through the nose the air we breathe out, as well as through the bowels the waste material we no longer need.

The end point on the Large Intestine official therefore lies, not where we might expect it from our knowledge of Western medicine, in the region of the bowel, but at the nose, at a point called Welcome Fragrance. In this name alone lies an indication of the Large Intestine's function of cleansing and purifying. It is also there to get rid of waste thoughts, stale impressions, ideas we have grown out of. It works very closely with the Small Intestine, to which it is physically attached, taking over the waste products of this official's activities and through its long convolutions wringing every drop of goodness from what the Lung has taken in, the Stomach has processed and the Small Intestine has sifted, before eliminating the remainder. Both Lung and Large Intestine are closely connected with ensuring the purity of all the other officials' work.

Grief, like the element whose emotion it reflects, is a hidden emotion. It is not one we can easily share, as we can joy, or even one we can easily observe, like anger. It feeds on the depths within us, and requires quiet and space of those around it. It is an expression of loss, of something from which we are cut off, shut out, and the thing lost, whatever the shape of that loss, preoccupies us, preventing us from moving forward. It can obsess us so that for the remainder of our life the shadow it casts over us hides the sunlight from us and we are unable to flourish or move on. It is with a weight of longing for what has gone before, never to return, that Metal people are burdened.

Where grief remains in balance, it will dominate our feelings for a while as we try to come to terms with it. It could be said that we need time to make meaning of such loss, time to find a context in which to place it. We can grieve for many things, for a child we have lost, or a child we can never bear or a love we can never be given, for the passing of something we had or the absence of something we yearn for. We can mourn a skill we will never gain, an aim we will always fail to achieve, an inadequacy in ourselves we can never dispel, as much as those things we have had which have now slipped from our grasp, and the sadness these bring is often more profound for it may not be leavened by some memory, however brief, of a past achievement.

And this feeling of loss may have particular poignancy in relation to that person who helped create us, our birth father, but who handed us over to our mother to nurture. Earth people, as we have seen, may feel that their mother has not nourished them. Metal people, on the other hand, may experience a feeling of loss in relation to their father, as though he has cut himself off from them. And they will feel the need deep within themselves to re-establish this lost connection. If a father is unable to enter into a close relationship with his child, that child will experience this rejection as an attack upon its own sense of self-value. Metal feels diminished in its own eyes if other people do not give it the respect it craves. Since it judges all things by its value, it will judge other people's feelings towards it in terms of how much these people value it. This differs from Fire, which will judge other people's feelings in terms of the love they are allowed to offer them.

Metal's need is to make sense of things, to see in them either significance and insignificance. It holds the judgement scales in its hand and will judge itself and others harshly and, when in balance, acutely. It is an intolerant element, but its intolerance is of a different kind from Wood's. Wood is irritated if people's actions run counter to what it sees as necessary, Metal is irritated by the inability of others to act or assess things appropriately. It is not there to act but to judge. Its task is to see the world in its true colours.

So serious is its task, so important is the speed with which it has to be carried out that Metal has no time to waste, for autumn's colours fade quickly and it has to work with death already in the air. If it does not do its work properly, the whole cycle of activity which precedes it will be as nothing, fading away like the autumn leaves trodden to dust underfoot. It is thus an impatient element, quick to judge, critical of others and above all of itself, incessantly seeking to unearth meaning from what lies buried within Earth's abundance. Most fully a yin element, it continues the inward-turning movement started by Earth, taking Earth's fruit and grinding it into ever tinier fragments, small enough to seep into the soil and into the air around us as the oxygen which gives us life. With this element we are at the furthest point from Wood and Fire's outward-turning energy.

Patrick, Proust and Presley

How, then, does this rarefied element manifest itself in flesh and bone in those whose signature it bears? Here I turn as example to my patient, Patrick. My interaction with him is a much more delicate affair than that which I have with the other patients I have so far described. Initially, before he and I got to know each other, I was on my mettle, as though under a spotlight. Setting such high standards for itself, Metal can be intolerant, too, of its practitioner, staying loyal only as long as this person can retain its full respect. He looked me over carefully and I felt as though it was I not he who was under intense scrutiny during this first meeting. I must have passed muster according to the criteria he set, for he has returned willingly for treatment. Of all the patients I have used here as example he is the most aware of what treatment does for him, almost immediately registering the changes he feels in himself, so acute is his judgement.

He has been a patient of mine for seven years. When he first came, I could not quite fathom what he wanted help with, almost as if he wasn't even sure himself why he had come. I can now see this as stemming from a deep inability to know who he was and what his life was about. This is a far cry, the furthest cry of all, from the very specific, so clearly spelt out needs expressed by James, my Wood patient. Treatment has changed this. Now if I ask Patrick why he comes to me, he is very clear in his response. He says that he now knows exactly where he is going, what his life is about and what he wants for the future for himself and his family. He sees treatment as continuing to give him inner clarity and maintaining a hard-won balance. We talk little during treatment, both of us quite clear as to his needs, each treatment consolidating what he has learnt about himself. Of all the patients I have treated this week, Patrick demands the most from me in terms of my insights and at the same time the least in terms of what I need to offer him if he accepts that these insights are appropriate.

Unlike my Earth patient, Andy, Patrick is sparse and to the point in his comments, arriving at the treatment with much that he wishes to discuss with me already processed and ready to be conveyed, where with Andy it is the activity of formulating his words which is the focus of his attention. Andy needs to involve me in the processing of his thoughts whereas Patrick wishes to share with me his insights into the conclusions he has already drawn and to assess them against what I have to offer. As he has done most of the work before arriving for treatment, I have to be quick in following his train of thought, and unlike Andy, he welcomes any intervention which adds to his understanding of things, and particularly of his understanding of himself and his place in life.

The demands he makes of me are ones he makes of himself. Once he had assured himself that what I offered him as acupuncturist was of value, he and I have settled into a very easy, but respectful relationship, where we value what each of us has to offer, I valuing his deep insights into himself and he valuing my skill in translating these insights into effective treatment. In that sense, once the initial, always prickly first interchanges between a Metal patient and his/her practitioner have been concluded satisfactorily, Metal is the easiest element to treat, for once it has assured itself of the practitioner's ability to understand the deep level of self-awareness and the need for self-respect and respect for others which any Metal person requires it makes little demands upon its practitioner.

If I compare Patrick with my other patients, I see that James (Wood) willingly handed control of the treatment over to me once he had convinced himself that what I have to offer was what he wanted. Rebecca (Fire) welcomes my interventions as proof of the good relationships we have set up between us. Both Andy (Earth) and now Patrick (Metal) to a greater extent ask to be allowed to dictate the terms of their encounter with me. My function here is somewhat more passive, as befits the more yin aspects of their respective elements.

Turning now towards the outside world for an example of the Metal element all of us can recognize, I am interested in how many famous faces spring immediately to mind. This is perhaps evidence of how it is the element which in many ways aspires most to a life lived at the highest level possible, public recognition being then one of the tokens of its achievements. The world of aspiration in its many guises (from the Latin word for in-breath), so Metal an activity, beckons temptingly to all Metal people. I could have chosen from amongst many that sprung to my mind, but in the end decided upon just two, a truly great writer and a truly great singer, the writer first, as representing the intake, the inspiration, the performer next, as representing the outbreath, the exhalation, Marcel Proust and Elvis Presley.

No greater example can be found of the Metal element manifesting so purely than in Marcel Proust, whose work encapsulates in the title of his greatest work all the longings a Metal person experiences. Translated word for word, it means 'In search of lost time', a meaning lost in the current translation, which I see is 'Remembrance of things past'. Translator that I was in another incarnation, I know that 'recherche', search, has about it the element of striving which is behind all Metal's activities, which 'remembrance', a much more passive activity, does not. And Proust himself, Metal to the last drop of his soul, lived immured in an airless room for much of his later life, racked by asthma, lost in contemplation of what might have been, a man from the past for whom that past became a total obsession, recoverable only in the many volumes of his book. Originally he wrote an unsatisfactory sketch for the book in the first person, and only found his true voice when he detached himself from himself, as it were, by re-writing the book, this time in the third person, as though looking at himself from afar. This gave him the necessary distance which Metal people need from which to assess his life and his experiences, the subject-matter of his whole work. By placing themselves at one remove from what they experience, they gain a perspective to assess the truth of what they observe.

It is the Metal element, therefore, which is the most capable of making a detached appraisal of what is going on, and Metal people are the best people from whom to ask advice, for, seeing things with a clarity other elements can only envy, they will sum the situation up in a few succinct words, almost coldly and mercilessly, and then move away, impatient if you show signs of not seeing as clearly as they do. When they are involved themselves, though, this clarity may become blurred by their own fears and needs, and then they, too, may be unable to see things for what they are, exaggerating these as all elements do when imbalances make them lose their own sense of perspective.

A different kind of detachment can be seen in our next example, that of Elvis Presley. And here, rather than locking himself in a room to write, we see someone who dwelt in the public gaze, but nonetheless in some profound way hid himself behind an aura of untouchability quite apparent when he was on stage. All performers require something from their audiences, for this need must lie behind their wish to perform in public. How such a need expresses itself will differ widely depending on the individual performer. We have seen that Billy Connolly enjoys the warm interaction with his audience that Fire demands of all around, and that Princess Diana, in her very differing way, had a deeply felt desire to surround herself with an audience offering the warmth and support which Earth craves. Here, with Elvis, we see another need expressed, that for a kind of adulation from his audience, but one which differs from that which Billy Connolly so obviously enjoys. Both appear to us on stage, the one warmly engaging with his audience, the other standing as though isolated in the stage lights, a lonely figure in the midst of all those grasping and frantic hands reaching out to him. And, however close they were to him, sometimes even pulling at him, the hands at some level did not seem to reach him, although they may have touched him physically. He seemed to have built for himself an invisible glass cage on the stage, creating a space around himself, a reflection, I feel, of how Metal at some deep level would dearly love to live in its own private, inviolate world. And yet, and here is the ambiguity which all elements hide within themselves, it was only through the admiration of others that Elvis could satisfy his search for self-respect, asking millions to offer him what he found difficult to offer himself.

All three, Elvis, Diana and Billy, in their differing ways need or needed an audience. They thrive by living in the limelight, and yet the light this casts over them has a different hue. We feel we are on the stage with Billy and become engaged with him in everything he does, our mutual laughter and joy forming a bridge across which we reach out to each other. Diana's relationship with us was more complex. She seemed to relish the presence of observers, and yet there remained something more of a distance between us than there is with Billy. We observe her but do not participate with her, a little unsure of what she wants of us. With Elvis we withdraw even further, our interaction with him now reduced to a minimum, our mere presence sufficient witness to the aura he cast around him, with no further contact between us demanded by him except the homage we are paying him as we watch.

He stands supremely alone on the stage, performing as though according to some inner ritual, aware of all those around him, but not allowing them to infringe upon his space. He wears brilliant white suits, studded with bright metal objects, a gleaming pure vision before us. He is a picture of extremes, black hair, black eyes, black brows, white suit, white shoes, pale face. His music, too, reflects a longing for what has never been, bearing within it all the pain of the world, all its loss. It weeps for what he longs for and cannot achieve. And this longing is for what lies beyond him, for all that he cannot reach, echoing perhaps his longing for his natural father, whom he lost to prison when he was a tiny child and for all the acting achievements in good film parts which he felt were denied him. And in true Metal fashion he tried to replace his lost father with a mentor who led him further astray, forcing him to accept parts in worthless films, further feeding his deep loss of self-respect. And yet at his death, steeped in drugs, living what he himself considered a worthless life, he was reading books on ancient Chinese philosophy. And how sad yet appropriate that there was so little left of value within him at the time of his death that he should have been found dead upon the lavatory, that symbol of all the waste we expel from our bodies. How he would have hated this final indignity.

When removed from the glamour of the public eye, his was a tragic life. Throughout it he had glimpses of the heights Metal always seeks to achieve and yet he let himself be seduced by lesser gods and the false coin of those surrounding him. His is indeed an extreme example of the Metal element's dilemma. It seeks only the pure and the noble and the worthwhile, and if it fails in this quest it may, in an act of almost wilful self-abnegation, instead have to make do with the impure, the ignoble and the worthless. Its gleaming gold can become buried deep beneath thick layers of mud and dirt, hidden from its deepest self. No other element suffers such an extreme challenge, always potentially an Icarus aiming for the stars only to fall when its wings fail.

My Metal element shadow

As I complete my look at what the Metal element brings to us, it is appropriate now that I use my own Metal element to take stock of what I was hoping to achieve when I started writing this book. This is the kind of act of self-appraisal which Metal people engage in all the time, but usually more privately than I am doing here. One of my aims in writing, I now realize, though it was not initially so obvious to me, was to clarify my own thoughts so that it was by working my way through the different facets of my practice that each has become a little more transparent to me. I had first to work out the perspective from which I wanted readers to view things. Was it to be from the viewpoint of a practitioner or from that of someone quite unfamiliar with acupuncture? How much detail would it be good to give? I was concerned that the examples I gave for famous people I considered good illustrations of the different elements might make too stereotyped than they are our perceptions of how the elements manifest themselves in all their uniqueness within each one of us. Examples are necessarily always inadequate, especially when they relate to the infinite complexities of the human being, but I felt we needed some that were common to most readers to give a firmer basis to the necessarily somewhat crude over-simplifications with which I lace my descriptions of the elements and to ground in the here and now much that might appear so abstract.

Looking back, as the Metal element always does if it is to evaluate for itself how far I have achieved my objective here, I feel pleased that I have written something that gives, to me, a true flavour of some of the depths of my practice and of the elements which underpin it. Again, my Metal element remains dissatisfied with whatever I do, as at some level it almost must, for it seeks the perfect, and perfection is an impossibility, and it is therefore constantly critical of what I have written, scratching away at a sentence here, a thought there, deleting a chapter, frowning at some inadequate expression, trying to make what I write more complete, more accurate, rather than the inadequate approximation I often feel it to be. However much I work away at what I am writing, when I return to it I always feel there is something more I should add, some deeper meaning I could extract, and in this I recognize how far my two Metal officials influence me, as my Lung, longing always to open itself up to take in new thoughts, forces my Large Intestine to let at least part of them go to waste, else it will allow no room for further thoughts and other visions to come to me.

At some point, then, my Metal element will have to be brave enough to let this book go, sending it out into the world with my blessing, and in the hope that it will be understood for what it is, a serious attempt to add something to our understanding of ourselves and of our troubling uniqueness.

And whilst I look at what my Metal officials offer me here, what have the other three elements we have looked at so far done to help me in this task? My Wood element, I see, has worked hard to plan the book, structure the sentences, organize the chapters, decide how and when to get it printed and make sure that in this long process I do not give up hope where, at intervals, hopelessness and feelings of my own inadequacy threatened to overwhelm me. My Fire element, closest of all to me, compelled me to share these thoughts with others, in an attempt to share with my readers my joy in my work, with my Small Intestine, my own personal territory among the officials, labouring daily at the task of sifting and sorting, sifting and sorting. My Earth element has helped me process all these myriad ideas whirring away in my mind, and interestingly, too, during the time of the book's gestation I found it difficult to feed myself, relying instead on others to do this or forgetting to feed myself, for all my attention was upon another form of processing altogether, not of my body but of my thoughts. And we have seen what my Metal officials contributed, and how hard they have had to work, particularly as I near the end of my writing, as I force myself to delete cherished words or unclear thoughts.

And finally, then, you may be wondering when I will get round to the last element, Water, an element I feel almost reluctant to approach, so in awe am I of its ephemeral nature, its insubstantiality, and at a certain level also somewhat afraid of its depth and its power, that I feel mere words cannot do it justice. I have left it to the last, but it could just as well have been the first, for with Water the elements draw together, become one, a flowing, unbroken circle of energy encompassing all within their grasp. With bated breath, then, the gift of my Metal element to my final work here, I move on to Metal's child, with which to complete the cycle. And here I need to tread delicately or, perhaps better, float gently, using as light a touch as I can for in Water only light things can float. I hope that I can find the words to do justice to this most mysterious of all elements, as we sink gently down into the cold of winter, and attempt to explore the darkness out of which all things, and each of our lives, emerge.

CHAPTER 9

THE WATER ELEMENT

Imperceptibly autumn has given way to the cold, and I have my first glimpse of winter here on the plains of Northern France as I approach Paris by train. The deadness of the land is more visible as I speed through the flatness of the country. A layer of white hoar frost lies over everything, surprisingly different from the warmer English countryside. This white haze, stretching as far as the eye can see, starts to draw the different shapes of the landscape into a whole which no other season does. That stark individuality of the autumn landscape it is replacing gave no such indication of unity. Instead, it seemed to emphasize individual differences, the shades of one tree in the same wood and of the same variety as its neighbours standing starkly out against the similar but always subtly different shading of its neighbours.

Now here, with a morning mist suddenly obliterating the landscape, for one brief moment train, country and I are swallowed up into one single unit, at one with each other in the midst of this white glow. When the mist dispersed, as it did after a few moments, the flat whiteness that spread over all that was around me enveloped me once more. Things looked as though pressed tight to the ground, even the moving objects, the cars and people I saw on the roads alongside, seeming to be swallowed up, made still, by the sheen of frost covering them.

The ground looks hard and flat, no living thing growing upon it, all things as though pressed down within it. The heaviness of the frost makes immobile each covered branch, standing translucent against the pale blue morning sky. The sun shines, but weakly, low on the horizon even at this late morning time. A pond we pass is covered in a shimmer of ice. The eye wanders far, unhindered by leaf and flower, the branches bare and stark. The morning light, herald of a bright day, is cold and chill, harbinger not of heat to come, but of a lessening of the cold. There is something bleached about the sunlight, too, as if life has leached out of it, bled it whiter and dryer. There is a paleness to all things, unleavened, as the land will be in deepest winter, by the sharp contrasts which deep snow in its purity and brilliance throws up.

Now the warmth in the carriage is welcome, distancing me from the arduous life winter outside demands of us. The window between us, keeping the warmth in and the cold out, cocoons me, makes me feel safe as I watch the winter world flow past outside its protective wall. I can only dimly imagine my body's response if I were to step out from this warmth into the cold of the winter landscape. Sitting here, I feel my cheeks tingle and shrink, my body draw towards itself in sympathy, as it anticipates the feeling of chill which would strike its pores, a transient reminder of the threat of cold.

Something of danger always seems to be in the air as the cold starts to seep into me, a feeling that I must be on my guard lest I am caught unawares without shelter outside. We hurry indoors, afraid to linger too long in this unfriendly environment. Though the clarity and beauty of a winter's day awes me, its purity strips things bare, makes them seem extreme in their starkness. In our attempts to protect ourselves against the cold we engage in some primitive fight for survival, with none of the ease the summer months bring us. And though summer, too, is extreme, shrivelling us with its heat, it only needs a little protective shelter and a few drops of water for us to survive. But here in winter I must arm myself with much greater protection, hidden outside beneath layers of warm clothing, every part of me except my face huddled against the cold, drawing myself with relief into the shelter of closed

doors and comfortable central heating, and heading for my
well-stocked freezer whenever I need food.

Metal has given a further twist to the wheel of the
elements, each in turn completing its task before handing on
its achievements and failures, a continuous and endless channel
through which life passes on its way towards eternity, each
element a prayer-bead slipping slowly through the hands of
time. And the thread along which these beads are strung is held
softly, but tenaciously, in the flowing hands of the last and most
mysterious of elements, Water, with which our journey, like
everything else that finds its way into its watery grasp, comes
full circle. For Water is the great unifier, drawing all things, not
to a close, but to a closed circle, in its great strength refusing to
allow even mountain-ranges to stand in the way of its quest for
unity, and slicing drop by drop relentlessly but with apparent
gentleness both through hard rock-face and soft sand, until it
finds its way back to itself.

Metal, the most ethereal of all elements, seeking to extract
the pure from the dross of life, gives way in turn to the last
element of the cycle, Water, more mysterious even than the
mysteries of life buried within Metal's breast, for Water is
the alpha and omega of all, both the end of the cycle of the
year in winter, and the point of its rebirth in the next spring.
Water is the hidden element, difficult to diagnose, often
misdiagnosed, because of its hidden, most yin nature. All
hides in winter, cowers down below ground to survive, and
all Water people convey this quality of hiddenness, of ultimate
unknowability. Somehow we are uneasy in the presence of a
Water person, unsure of them, as they are of themselves. There
is an elusiveness to Water which no other element possesses,
the absolute opposite of the supreme knowability of a Wood
person who is so obviously there foursquare in front of us.

It is useful to picture each element in terms of their physical
presence in this way. Both Wood and Fire are yang, out there
in their visibility, Wood, having the clearest contours of all, a

little starker than Fire's. By contrast, Earth's outline seems to grow a little more blurred, a little more yin, Metal's boundaries are more immaterial, imbued with a little more of the spirit, and Wood's more material, more of the physical body. With Water we reach the most immaterial of all, so blurred in outline that in grasping a handful of water it eludes our fingers drop by drop, or, even more insubstantial, transforms its very nature into steam or ice to escape us further.

Water's needs are diffuse, less focused upon the individual, for with Water we enter a boundless world, so different from that bounded territory which emerges from within itself as the buds of Wood. Here we reach the most yin depths of the cycle of life, where things merge and flow into one another, their edges blurred, their individual forms so indistinct that a person swimming in the ocean is rendered almost invisible by the immense expanse in which he floats. We can barely lift our heads above the waves, so strong is the pull from below, and despite efforts to stay afloat will eventually be drawn under to merge like some individual drop with all the other drops forming this immensity. Where each bud declares its presence in clear outline, a statement of emerging individuality, the drops of water which are the Water element's contribution to the cycle of life lose their contours as they touch each other, flowing together into one vast expanse. Here the individual significance which Metal works so hard to seek for itself is submerged beneath the cover winter spreads over all things. In winter and in Water everything becomes one, held in a tight embrace. The individual can survive only by clinging to the others around, as all things cower down together. The cycle of the elements comes full circle, Water its end and its beginning, drawing all things into a spiral out of which Wood will then emerge once more as the start of the new cycle.

The shapes of Water

Each element holds within itself the knowledge of its own and special secret, that particular gift of which it is the unique trustee, and to which no other element has the key. For Wood, it is the ability to start, for Fire the ability to relate, for Earth the ability to sustain, and for Metal the ability to extract. Water's special gift is the ability to rejoin. In Water there echoes the profound and age-old memory of a time when all things were one, before the universe burst outwards into existence, flinging matter far out into the furthermost reaches of space. It was Water's eternal flow and rhythm which gradually shaped the world, existing as it did before Earth was born, before sun, moon and stars lit up the skies and warmed the seed of Man sufficiently to coax him into existence inside that very microcosm of the original unity of the universe, the watery bed of his first cell.

The great wheel of the elements, endlessly turning, rests in turn upon one of its five spokes, each a moment in the cycle from birth to death and on to birth again. And each turn of the wheel echoes the rise and fall of life, the moment of birth finding the little bud of Wood peering hopefully out of the dead land into the new world of spring, before calling upon Fire's warmth to ripen it to maturity. And on the wheel turns, bearing with it the fruit of Fire's labours to drop into Earth's ample bosom as food to sustain life, where Metal, watching from afar, swoops down to extract one bright and pure and precious jewel worthy of bearing on high.

The moment at which Metal soars upwards to the skies above is the point of our greatest detachment from the whole, the peak of our individuality. Metal stands alone with its precious prize, so dearly won, proud of its great achievement but in the sad knowledge of its futility, for that very prize contains within it the seed of death. And ironically, but appropriately, as all things must be, as the wheel turns gently on to float in Water, Metal's great yearning to regain its lost paradise is effortlessly answered, for Water bears within it that knowledge of paradise regained so desperately and vainly sought by Metal. We have reached the moment in the cycle where we merge ourselves in the whole again, drawn down into the watery depths of all that is. As the waters reclaim us we thankfully yield ourselves to them, reduced once more by their gentle but unyielding force to abandon all attempts at soaring up.

Water's eternal ebb and flow, grinding the rock of our individuality to dust and sucking us back down to merge like droplets in the ocean, makes a mockery of our attempts to be ourselves. Arrogantly individual as we reach Metal, we are now taught the hardest and most ambiguous lesson of all, that we are worth nothing. Nature, like all great Masters, stands above us, as we boast of our achievements in our ignorance, and knocks us back down into Water's remorseless grasp, wordlessly teaching us humility. We can drown, attempting to fight its great currents, or humbly learn to accept its power, sinking back into the undifferentiated whole again, at one with our fellows, no more, no less than any floating at our sides.

Winter is Water's season. All things cower down to survive its bitter cold, huddling together, like those droplets in the ocean, to find protection in bulk against the harsh conditions outside. The land opens its arms and pulls inside it all it can lay hold upon, the trees and bushes, cleared of unnecessary leaves, sinking lower and sending all their vitality and strength deep into their roots to guard against extinction. The time at which the year sinks from autumn into winter requires of us the greatest courage. As the cold, harsh days pass slowly by, we cannot know whether we have amassed sufficient strength to survive until spring. It is the time when nature has to trust the most to its own powers of regeneration, for that wheel, turning now slowly and laboriously over the icy wastes against the force of the storms, may falter and grind to a halt if the bleak winter winds howl and scream too harshly against it.

Now we will discover whether Nature's busy work in gathering together its reserves has been sufficient, before winter's cold curtain descends over the land. The year has yielded all it can, and forces us to call a halt. Winter offers us a pause to catch our breath after the heavy labours of the year, and we must welcome it as such, gratefully receiving the peace of inaction that it offers us, for without a time to withdraw within ourselves we would become exhausted.

No individual creation can withstand Water's inexorable progress as it rolls over the dead and humbled land, but that act of bowing our head to its implacable authority can become in our hands a gesture of humiliation, or of splendid triumph. Where Metal's achievements have failed to yield the essence of pure and rare things worthy of winter storage within the heart of each individual watery cell, winter will represent a time of defeat, turning what should become an interval of quiet and passive contemplation into a watery grave, wherein lie buried the bones of the future. But whatever Metal has held triumphantly aloft will become the past's cherished legacy to the future, helping us rise again like some triumphant phoenix from the ashes of our past mistakes. And these things Water clasps to itself in its deep oceanic sleep, allowing their subtle presence to enrich and nourish as trace elements of future growth.

Down from the outermost reaches of space Water has floated, combining, condensing and endlessly changing shape and form before spreading itself in a film upon the face of the earth to become the seed-bed of all life. Over the torn and bleeding surface of this planet, blown to its lonely resting-place in space, it lays a gentle and healing hand, soothing its weary brow, flattening its mountains, raising its valleys and moving its continents, trying with all the power in its possession, and great indeed is Water's power, to mould Earth's contorted and scarred surface into a beautiful and flowing whole. Endlessly repairing the tears and rents in the canvas of the universe torn by that first cataclysmic explosion, its deft fingers busily stitch and sew, drawing together and spreading apart. Lovingly, and for what great purpose we may only dimly perceive, it prepares the land to receive the great gift of life, for it is the medium through which everything passes on its way to becoming alive.

Wherever it encounters obstacles to its own smooth ebb and flow, there it must set to work, passively and indifferent to all but its own absorbing need to envelop and smooth away whatever it finds deflecting its great and unifying tide. All it wants is to be left in peace to be itself, drifting and floating at one with its fellows in the billowing ocean of all that is, and for this right it will work hard and long, silently but inexorably fighting its eternal battle to force into defeat whatever gets in its way. A master of disguises, it has learnt to don a multiplicity of masks, evading capture by transforming itself under the very eyes of its captors. Fleeing alike the summer's heat and winter's freezing breath, it will abruptly change its watery home to live elusively amongst misty vapours or defended by barriers of solid ice whenever it feels threatened by extinction, biding its time and awaiting the moment when it can return to its watery shape again. Like some eternal cuckoo, it will make its home wherever it finds itself, gracefully and with ease taking up new residence amongst both icy wastes and misty clouds.

Apparently passive and lazy, it offers no resistance to the endless buffetings of wind and cold and heat, emerging victorious where less flexible elements would long since have succumbed, its very passivity proving its strength. By itself each of those tiny and insignificant drops together forming the great oceans of the sea and the billowing clouds of the air is too weak to survive such onslaughts, but banded together with its fellows it becomes a terrifying opponent against which all the might of the other elements is as nothing. If allowed the freedom to flow as it wishes, Water will become life's soothing and merciful companion, bringing harmony and wholeness to all it touches. All life is awash with its energy, as it flows through our veins and floods our cells, but under threat this life-giving force can overwhelm and destroy, consigning Wood's hopeful buds to a soggy death, reducing Fire's warmth to spluttering embers, flattening the Earth and drowning Metal's precious gifts fathoms deep.

A raging torrent one moment, a stagnant puddle the next, held tight in a glacier's cruel grasp or floating softly down in the morning dew, it has the power to be all things to all men, but in so being fears that it may be nothing in particular to itself. Its very changeability safeguards it from destruction, endowing it with the special gift of endless transformation, and yet its own instability and unpredictability frighten it, for even less than Earth does it know where it is at any moment, for the next may well find it elsewhere. Burdened with the insecurity of knowing that it is incapable of remaining in any shape for long enough to make it its home, it will crave the peace of inertia and stillness, its attempts at rejoining itself an endless and unsatisfied search for rest.

Earth has no power to transform itself away from its long-established and comfortable presence below our feet, but Water never knows where its next home will be, forever and necessarily unstable, that instability bestowing upon it both the comforting gift of survival and the endless terror of knowing that but one brief moment's isolation from its companions is sufficient to render it powerless, a single and insignificant raindrop abandoned on a leaf to be brushed away indifferently by the merest breath of wind or evaporated by the first rays of the morning sun.

Where Earth, its lifelong companion, would dearly love to learn the lesson of motion from Water's flowing hands, Water looks yearningly for stability to Earth's enduring presence. Having been given the gifts of restlessness, movement and change as the powerful weapons with which it fights for its life, its great longing is for the courage to rest motionless, inert and unchanging wherever it chooses. For in the stagnant pools and murky puddles there lies lurking, sombre and still, Water's shadow-side tempting it to detach itself from its fellows and lie down alone to sleep. And therein lies Water's downfall, for once it allows itself to be lured to a standstill it becomes a prisoner, forever condemned to lifeless stagnation, forgetting that it possesses the great gift of transformation with which to escape its fate.

Water fears that it may become detached from the comforting arms of the whole to stand powerless, lonely and alone. Its great terror is that it will drown in its own individuality. Its great learning is to find the courage fearlessly to allow itself, companionless, to be itself, not a lifeless dreg abandoned on the bottom of a stagnant pool, but a single teardrop proudly bearing within itself all the joys and sorrows of life.

Water shapes us, as it shapes all things. It is the flow and rhythm of life's sap within us. Guided by the structure and definition of the other elements, its great tide is channelled into the narrow confines of our cells, the delicate arteries of our blood and all the myriad pathways of fluid which feed our hormones and our tears. Only with Water's indomitable force can life be lived, and thus it is our will to survive. Those living their lives showered with its blessings will bear the imprint of its implacable strength. Apparently bending to the whim of all who bear upon them, yet they make their own will prevail, echoing the inexorable progress of flood water as it drowns the land.

And yet, strong and brave as is this element, buried far beneath its flowing surface there lies within it an echo of that terror of the deep which we all feel, and fear is thus Water's companion, where joy lights Fire's way, for might we not drown in those depths? Its colour is the blue of the ocean, its body bears the sharp smell of stagnant water and the sound of its voice can be the hesitant gurgle of a stream finding its way between the rocks of a river bed, or the monotonous and far-distant murmur of the sea. Its two organs are the Kidney and the Bladder. As the waters of the world wash through and over us, they are drawn to us by the Kidney and passed through each cell by the Bladder's action. The Kidney, the storehouse of the very essence of our life, creates the cells out of which life develops, each embryo lying kidney-shaped in the womb.

And so the great cycle restarts, as the tiny seed nestles deep down in its watery bed awaiting the warmth of spring to draw its shoots up into the daylight of a new life.

Alex and David Beckham

What kind of person lives their life under this often harsh guardian, subject to extremes and forced to adopt all manner of disguises to survive? What imprint does this constant shadow of fear place upon those with Water as their element?

Something of elusiveness is in all Water people, a quality hard to define since its very purpose is to render those displaying it in some way invisible, and thus to enable them to hide. Water's movements always have about them some of the fluidity of a cat's, with an ability to slip silently away from us. And of all the elements it is Water which has the most to gain by masking itself, those bearing its mark echoing the many ways Water adapts itself in nature for a similar purpose. They can freeze as animals do when cornered, they can boil over, their fury unequalled even by the hard anger of Wood or the cutting anger of Metal, or, when at their most comfortable, meander at ease, if no impediment hinders their smooth progress, allowing us then, too, to feel at ease in their presence. Water is the toughest element of all, still there when all the other elements have given up, and yet apparently at times frozen by the fear which is its emotion, like a rabbit caught in headlights.

There is thus within Water people an intangible, elusive quality which indicates their ability to change and hide from us, always some feeling emanating from them that creates slight wariness in us, as though, like them, we are unsure of how long they will remain as they are, and how far we can rely upon them to be as they present themselves to us now.

This elusive quality is present in my last patient, Alex, an uneasy yet tough person, one whom I would choose if I were to say which of all the patients I have so far looked at I could guarantee would survive come what may. Disasters often befall her, she gets herself into one difficulty after another, indeed appears almost to court disaster, losing money badly one minute, rich the next, panic-struck when things turn difficult, and yet always, always, bobbing up like the cork on the water that she will remain all her life just as I think she is on the point of going under.

She came for treatment for a bad lower back problem and frequent panic attacks. These were preventing her from doing what Water wants most to do, flow smoothly through life, like a brook babbling merrily along downstream, passing boulders and obstacles effortlessly on its journey to the sea. The feelings of panic were caused by periods in her life when the uncertainty which Water senses as underlying all things would surface, and though these recur less often since she has come for treatment she still needs me to reassure her that all will be well and that she will, as it were, survive the rigours of winter come what may. Her treatment appears to offer her a feeling of safety, the reassuring familiarity of our communion together. I find myself talking, not to her or at her, but with her, my voice a soothing accompaniment to what she is telling me. When I listen to us talking together, I hear our voices melding, as though flowing together along a stream of words. With no other element do I feel such gentle and continuous participation is welcome.

In her life she shows that determination to rise to the top which is Water's hallmark. There is a ruthlessness to all that she does, well hidden but always present, a drive to get where she wants to go whatever the obstacles before her. And yet this determination can be disguised by an apparent softness which often gives others the misguided feeling that she is malleable and easy to manipulate. This, so unlike the hard edges of Wood or Metal, enables her to deflect attack much as the martial artist learns to do, with almost imperceptible adjustments to position and approach, creating a yielding form of counter-attack. When out of balance she can flounder aimlessly, or stay becalmed, and yet that pull to survive is usually strong enough to enable her eventually to get herself afloat once more.

When I turn to look in the outside world for people to illustrate the Water element, the faces of some well-known people come to my mind, as they did when I was discussing the Metal element, though for very different reasons, and yet it is only recently that I have discovered how widespread the presence of this element is amongst those who reach the top. This is because I now realize that in the past I have often overlooked those specific Water qualities more than I have done with any other element. To my satisfaction, I am growing increasingly confident in uncovering this most elusive of all elements, seeing more clearly now than ever before its quality of ruthlessness and unyielding pressure, hidden behind a softer mask. It appears malleable, but pulling against it or trying to get it to move in another direction is like trying to stem the tide.

Something of this quality is clearly there in my choice of a famous Water person, David Beckham, yet when you watch him you are perhaps as surprised as I continue to be at the position he has assumed as the world's most famous footballer. How can this apparently unassuming young man, with apparently very little in the way of obvious ambition and love of power, have forced his way upwards into the limelight as he has done and continues to do, even though now his footballing skills appear somewhat on the wane. There are many other footballers who play as good, if not better, football to whom not a hundredth of the press coverage is dedicated.

So where does his power to attract such visibility reside? And what makes me so sure that he is of the Water element?

First his voice. It is slightly strange, monotonous and hesitant, with a kind of whine within it. If I were to describe it, I would say that it has an oddly high drone. This is the groaning voice of Water. It is certainly not an easy voice to listen to, oddly at variance with his look of control and ease in front of the camera, and it reveals something surprising about him, jolting me each time I hear it. He starts hesitantly, taking a long time to get going, and like water in nature, appears to me to be like a stream blocked by obstacles and at last forcing its way through. I can think of no more obvious an example of Water's voice than this one.

And once I was alerted to his voice some years ago I started to watch his progress as a highly visible example of the Water element. He came on the scene first as a fairly junior member of Manchester United's team, then rose to form part of the England team, and appeared to fall from grace in that famous incident when he was dismissed from the field. I noted how despite the gravity of the situation he appeared to be in total control as he walked off, tightly held in, and then I watched how he dealt with the insults and opprobrium the world heaped on him, apparently unaffected by these, indeed stubbornly defying them. And up he went, from outcast to captain of the same English team, and then, in a final smooth move, as a result of some tenacious determination to get his own way, he managed to irritate his manager so much that he forced him to release him to move to the football team, Real Madrid, which was then considered to be the greatest in the world.

No smoother transition from low to high could be imagined, and each step along the way seemed inevitable. And yet, if asked, we would have to admit that we are still unclear as to what he himself did to get himself promoted to captain of England or released to join Real Madrid. It is not only that he was an amazing footballer. There are many amazing footballers who never become captains of their team, never become footballing icons or fight their way to the top, as he has so smoothly done. There is a drive within him to achieve the highest, and he chooses carefully the path he needs to plot to get there, determined to take his place not only among his equals but as the best of the best. Here we also see expressed that drive towards self-promotion which makes him a marketing man's dream.

At every point, from playing, to hairstyle, to dressing, to lifestyle, to wife, he forces himself to the public attention, turning himself into the most marketable athlete in the world and drawing to him the eyes of all. It was not only his footballing skills but his carefully controlled marketability which persuaded Real Madrid to bid for him. And here it is significant evidence of his elusive Water character that he chooses to change hair styles and clothes like a chameleon. All these changes are by his choice, for he apparently allows nobody to dictate how he should dress or look. Hardly have we grown used to his mohican hair style or his pigtail, before he cuts his hair short or in a different style to confound us all, and send the fashion world scurrying to emulate him. In clothing too, he defies all the rules, wearing sarongs one day, elegantly dressed the next, smoothly wearing style after different style, bedecked with jewellery like a woman, only to appear a few hours later dishevelled and unkempt in mud-spattered football gear. He has what appears to be an unashamed, almost feminine delight in new clothes, and is not embarrassed to strut like some peacock on the world stage, and yet he is as masculine as can be imagined behind this finery. Even in this he masks his masculinity by his femininity and his femininity by his masculinity, an almost androgenous person, a changeling, who appeals to all people, male or female, old or young, thrilling us by his unknowability.

In all that he does he eludes us, one step ahead of the pack and of us at any moment. I sense that this is why he fascinates so many people. He is not as good-looking as others, not as articulate or as obviously intelligent as some, and yet here he is on the front pages of every newspaper and magazine in the world. Somehow, and we are not quite sure how he made it happen, he forced his way to the top almost as though through no obvious action of his own, much like the hidden pressure of water from below will force a fountain to gush. And his movements, too, are fluid; there is a flow to his game which it is a delight to watch.

He also appears to possess the warmth and camaraderie of Water, at ease with his fellow professionals, retaining qualities of the ordinary bloke which endear him to us all. There is no apparent flaunting of his successes, or deliberate distancing of himself which Metal might do in an attempt to gain people's admiration and respect. He remains one of the pack, that drop of water in an ocean Water people always welcome. It is power not respect that he is looking for, and Water's power comes from secret sources. We could indeed describe him as someone with hidden depths, disguised by that rather bland but ambiguous smile and apparently easy presence.

And is his emotion fear? Perhaps he is an ideal example of its hidden quality, the ruthlessness with which, fearing his position to be endangered, he acted by so skilfully and so secretly stoking up his manager's antagonism that we could almost say that he engineered his own dismissal and inevitable transfer to Real Madrid by forcing Ferguson's anger to explode in a blow. And he took great care to be viewed apparently as the wronged person, a further sign of Water's determination to come out on top. On TV somebody once asked him whether he was anxious when he took the final penalty kick which would decide whether England could go to the World Cup. He replied baldly, 'No. That's what I practise so hard for.' This was not spoken in arrogance but with an utter conviction of his own power, allied to a refusal to show by the barest flicker, as he positioned himself behind the ball, that deep fear he must have felt, but would never admit to, that he might fail himself and the whole of the country. This is the force, that fear of submitting to fear, which drives Water onwards so that to contemplate failure would be too frightening a thing to do.

Our place in the circle

The brief journey round the elements with some of my patients as example has stirred different feelings within me, their practitioner, as I have passed from one element to the next. I have moved from a feeling of a kind of vigorous activity with James, through a time of joy and laughter with Rebecca, on to a slightly more challenging encounter with Andy, then to a quieter place within myself where I encounter Patrick, before finding myself somewhat unsure and unsettled again when writing about Alex. And now I can feel myself almost with relief coming back full circle again to the safe, known resting place of Wood, as winter starts to yield to spring once more.

Other practitioners will experience these elements quite differently, although we will all have some reactions in common, since they are universal symbols of human experience. But the extent of the differences we experience will depend upon qualities unique to each of us, and to our own personal experiences in our encounters with people of different elements. Some people will find Wood and Metal more difficult than I do, Fire or Earth easier. I know that my own life has led me to understand the first two elements more deeply than the others, whilst other practitioner friends of mine have more difficulty with them, but cannot fathom why I find my own element, Fire, often more puzzling than any other element.

And this points to one of the great problems in any therapy, the extent to which therapists have or have not resolved their own conflicts. What is not resolved may make us overlook an emotional need in the patient which we are unable to deal with ourselves. Translated into acupuncture terms, this might mean that an acupuncturist, unable to reconcile his or her own sense of loss in some area of his/her life, may prefer, unconsciously, not to see the grief of their Metal patient, because of the conflict grief arouses in them, and may therefore, just as unconsciously, interpret the emotion as lack of joy (Fire) or lack of anger (Wood) to avoid confronting their own imbalances.

The important thing is not that we deny our own reactions, but that we be aware of how far they may cloud our judgement. For example, for a long time I found myself overlooking the existence of the Wood element in my patients until I realized the extent to which I had not dealt with this element as manifested in my mother. Once understood and explored, my relationship to Wood, in others as well as in myself, has become one of a trusted, though sometimes difficult friend, as my encounter with James has shown. And I found, too, that my relationship with my mother improved as my perceptions of how the element Wood acted itself out in her deepened. Metal I feel at ease with, as though understanding deeply its qualities, probably because I have had great helpers who have had Metal as their element, and have gained immeasurably from their sureness of judgement and acuteness of understanding.

Each practitioner therefore has to follow a similar journey in their understanding of the elements, assessing their own reactions to the differing manifestations of the elements, highlighting where these are exaggerated or defensive, and pinpointing where they have to make adjustments if they are to assess these elements' presence accurately in their patients. To some extent we can only see the elements through the lens of our own, for however much we try to clear our eyesight, making ourselves as neutral as possible, there always remains some slight patina of distortion when we look at other elements. The important thing is not to deny this, or even to bewail this fact, but to take this into account in every judgement we make so that we try to see our patient with eyes that are as unclouded as possible. That is why we need to know ourselves as deeply as possible before we can turn to helping others, and continue this work upon ourselves as we help them.

Such self-knowledge also implies that we have learnt ways of dealing with our own inadequacies and failings, have faced up to them and placed them in some context. Such a facing up to ourselves and acceptance of what we see within ourselves is how I define a state of balance. The pressures upon us from within and without mean that we constantly oscillate between balance and imbalance as we attempt to come to terms with what is demanded of us, and thus any state of balance presents a hard fight. During the time we are with our patients and in our judgements of them we must strive, however brief the time we are with them, (and in the timescale of our lives the few hours we are with our patients take up only a tiny part), to retain hold of that state of inner balance such an encounter demands of us.

The interrelationships of the elements within us one to another, with our own guardian element at their fulcrum, dictate our balance, and make us who we are. In the patient, too, the elements engage in their own dance of energy, but here the patient's task, unlike the practitioner's, is to use the practice room as the place in which the work required to move towards that desired state of self-knowledge is to be carried out. The practitioner acts as guide in this often troubling domain. To that extent practitioners must strive to leave outside the practice room those parts of themselves which may throw shadows over the patient and distort the true picture of the patient's needs. This is a challenging, yet ultimately deeply fulfilling, task.

Here again the elements come to help us, because our knowledge of them, honed with each year of practice, helps us not only help our patients but ourselves at the same time. If we are aware of how the elements manifest within ourselves both in and out of balance, we can draw upon this knowledge to understand what is going on not only within ourselves but in our interactions with our patients. Our own weaknesses and failings, as well as our strengths, always add to our practice, provided that we acknowledge them to ourselves, work on them, keep them always before our eyes as obstacles we may trip over, or chasms that may open up before our feet in the practice room. And each encounter offers a unique challenge, demands of us that we approach this person with fresh eyes, as far as possible place ourselves outside our own insecurities and worries, leaving behind as we enter the practice room all that may detract from that focused spotlight we play upon each patient.

And no element can be complete in itself. It depends upon the others as they depend upon it, just as autumn cannot make a year, nor remain autumn forever. Each element, each season, is only one segment of the complete cycle, forming part of a process which moves towards a completion it alone cannot achieve. And one element completes itself only by moving on to the next element, the culmination of its work becoming the point of transition to what comes next. Wood therefore achieves its fulfilment in Fire, Fire in Earth, and so on, as does spring in summer and autumn in winter.

And one way we find to help us complete ourselves will be in our choice of friends and partners. It is as though we often need to draw on the resources of others, with their different guardian elements, in order to find what we cannot find within ourselves, to round out, as it were, our own one-dimensional figure into the five dimensions of the elements. A Metal person, whose emotion is grief, may look to others to furnish himself with his emotional supply of joy, anger, sympathy or fear. A Wood person might look for the firm boundaries a Metal person is better able to provide. Our need to draw other emotions to us to offset our dominant emotion may encourage us to choose partners or friends of another element to support us in an area of the emotional spectrum which is alien to us. We may prefer to venture out into another

element's unfamiliar emotional territory in this way, with all
the attendant dissatisfactions and disturbances our intolerance
of each other's differences creates, even though it was those very
differences which prompted our original choice.

Each element will therefore need to call upon the qualities
of the other elements in other people to provide what we
ourselves lack. This is how we come to make all manner of what
may seem, to ourselves and others, to be surprising choices with
respect to our relationships, jobs and living situations. Often
without knowing it, we attempt to supplement something we
ourselves lack by reaching out for those qualities in those with
whom we choose to set up relationships of all kinds. It could
be said that we need each other for our differences as well as
for our similarities, even though we may ourselves be unaware
of this, and this is one of the reasons why we may fall in love
with people utterly unlike ourselves, or make choices of friends
we are ourselves puzzled by. In the apparently unlikely lovers
and friends we choose there are qualities which we recognize,
as though by instinct, as in some way complementing or
challenging our own.

For obvious reasons, the choices we make when we are out
of balance will differ greatly from those of our balanced state.
A Fire person, though needing the energy of a Metal person
to simulate and enhance him, may find these same energies
overwhelming if his own Fire energy has become weakened.
What may be right and beneficial when we are in balance can
become something far less appropriate when we are not. The
rounding off we hope from our relationships with others will
then become, instead, a diminishing, a lessening of ourselves.
And here we may not so much complement as further push
ourselves off balance. Our choices, taken from a position
of imbalance, may distort an already unbalanced situation.
Having already a low sense of self-esteem, for example, we
may choose as partner or friend somebody who delights in
belittling us, in our imbalance seeking out what is familiar

to us, rather than having the courage to find someone who sees a value in us which we are at that point unable to see. As we move towards balance, therefore, we will find our choice of relationships change as an increased feeling of self-worth encourages us to seek out those who respect us for who we are rather than those who choose to undermine our sense of self.

CLOSING THE CIRCLE

CHAPTER 10

A 21ST-CENTURY CONTEXT

Having circled the elements. What now? Throughout this book I have so far looked at acupuncture as though in isolation, a thing apart from the culture in which it is practised, but it is time to place it in some context in the world of medicine.

According to what we know at present, acupuncture appears to have originated in China some 2500–3000 years ago, and spread from there throughout the Far East, finally reaching the West a hundred years or more ago and in isolated instances a few centuries earlier. Its greatest impact here has been from the mid-1950s onwards and continues to grow. Its geographical spread, from the Far East to the West, and its spread over time, from the pre-Christian era to the 21st century, have built up 3000 years or more of accumulated knowledge, adding layer upon layer, in many languages and from many countries, to the original facts and skills which have come down to us from those ancient of days and ancient of places.

What I practise and teach in 21st-century London is therefore inevitably very different from what a Chinese acupuncturist would practise and teach in ancient China. What both of us have in common, as far as anybody can verify this at this vast distance in time, are the philosophical concepts upon which our practice is based, concepts such as the wholeness of all things, the Dao, the polarity inherent in this wholeness, known as yin and yang (as manifest in the polarity of health and ill-health), the cyclical phases, the five elements (as manifest in the passage of the seasons and the days), the concept of qi energy and its distribution through the body in pathways called meridians, and finally the understanding that the insertion of a needle into points along these meridians can affect health. There are, of course, many other points of similarity which I and my ancient Chinese counterpart have in common, and so far we would talk a common language.

There are, however, huge swathes of my practice which would puzzle him, as I would be puzzled by his needling technique or use of specific points. Equally, I will be puzzled by the introduction of herbs or a different method of moxibustion into the practice of a modern colleague trained in another branch of acupuncture, such as Japanese acupuncture or modern Chinese acupuncture, as they will be by my frequent use of moxibustion or my method of needle insertion.

To complicate the matter further, in recent years there have emerged further branches of acupuncture, often related to areas of Western medicine, such as physiotherapy or surgery, in which the link to ancient Chinese practice has been even more tenuous as to be almost invisible. Large philosophical concepts have made way for small concepts, such as local pain relief. Ear acupuncture is a case in point. You only need to know how to insert a needle, its insertion depth, and where to insert it to practise it, a matter of a few days' or even a few hours' basic training. The Dao and yin/yang, and the whole philosophical foundation which they underpin, have here disappeared without trace.

In addition to acupuncture, there are all those other practices which have allied themselves to the practice of inserting a needle: moxibustion, palpation, qi gong, tuina, breathing exercises, herbs, diet, to name but a few. According to your branch of acupuncture, one or other will probably have been included in your acupuncture practice at some point. This is similar to what happens in Western medicine, too, where different hospitals, different consultants within those hospital and different medical practitioners outside the hospital have their own treatment regimes for their patients. My doctor told me that a colleague recently admitted to the practice had been qualified at the same hospital as she had, and 'that means we speak the same kind of language'. Patients are offered physiotherapy, chemotherapy or counselling, or are told to take exercise or to diet. The kinds of exercise or physiotherapy will differ from hospital to hospital and surgery to surgery, as will the drugs prescribed and their prescription doses.

This is much like the situation prevailing in acupuncture. Different schools of acupuncture will lay a different emphasis on what they offer their patients. The five element acupuncturist, for example, tends to offer only acupuncture, moxibustion and lifestyle advice. Other branches of acupuncture will offer moxibustion, too, but their moxa cones may be smaller or larger, be placed on a needle or on a cone of ginger or originate in Japan rather than China. Yet other branches will use no moxibustion at all. The way I needle will be different from the action of a modern Chinese acupuncturist and a modern American acupuncturist. I'm sure all three of us would be amazed if we were to be transported back in time to watch an ancient Chinese acupuncturist needle with what are thought, perhaps fancifully, to be the original stone needles. This is akin to the astonishment with which a modern surgeon would watch surgery carried out 200 years ago.

To know where to insert a needle to effect some significant change in a patient's energy requires a knowledge of the basic philosophical concepts of the Dao, yin/yang, the five elements, the meridian system and qi energy. Without this knowledge, any insertion of needles may have a slight local effect, much as rubbing a sore spot helps the tenderness to disperse, but will not be able to produce the profound changes which represent true acupuncture. Brief, often merely month-long, courses in acupuncture are popular in the Western medical world because of their brevity, and, at a deeper level, I suspect, also because they appear to confirm that acupuncture is at heart something so essentially simple to learn that it cannot rival its Western counterpart. But these have nothing in common with the years of study required to achieve a true understanding of acupuncture's scope. And they do a disservice to all because they delude the unwary into equating acupuncture with a technical skill, easily acquired and simple in its reach, thereby depriving many of the chance to explore it further.

Where, then, do I see acupuncture's place amongst the many other forms of healing now practised? And, since we are discussing five element acupuncture here, we should look at it both within the context of physical medicine as we conceive of it in a Western context and of the wide spectrum of those other practices we can place under the broad banner of psychotherapy. The fact that we can do so is proof that acupuncture has been sufficiently flexible and universal to have developed its own particular Western focus, for what I practise can be said to correspond, among other things, and surprisingly closely, too, to the psychological advances the eras of Freud, Jung and their many successors have ushered in, but with its own special emphasis. This, coupled with its coherent approach to redressing physical ills, makes it particularly relevant to a modern society beset with very different stresses from those of two or more millennia ago. It is to acupuncture's credit that it has been able to adapt itself so magnificently to the changing needs of many different centuries and many different cultures, attesting thus to its universal significance.

I therefore like to feel that acupuncture's strong emergence in the West since the middle of the 20th century has about it something so right that it, too, confirms for me that pattern which for the ancient Chinese underlaid all things, for it has appeared at a time when we are coming to the end of an era of often mindless homage to Western medicine's reach, and are instead slowly, perhaps too slowly, starting to question the limits of that reach. It also comes at a time when the many discoveries of science have opened up to us as never before concepts about the forces moulding all things which run counter to much previously received scientific opinion on the nature of the physical universe. Matter now dissolves before our eyes into something remarkably close to what the ancient Chinese called qi energy, and the soul which resides within this body of ours is now accepted as affecting the world it looks out upon. The linking of all things, so clearly perceived by those ancient precursors of ours, now finds its confirmation in modern physics.

Only Western medicine appears to lag behind here, perhaps not surprisingly, for much about these new perceptions threatens many of the assumptions upon which it is based. And this is the challenge acupuncture faces, for in many profound ways it is far ahead of the field in terms of its understanding that all things form part of an indivisible whole. It has therefore been able to develop its understanding of what constitutes human health and what can be done to maintain or restore the balance of that health within a holistic context. Despite its antiquity, acupuncture remains truly a pioneer at the frontiers of a new approach to medicine, and by its very presence threatens a medical status quo so entrenched as to feel almost impregnable in its resistance to new ideas.

The irony is that something as old as the hills should also be as new as the latest scientific advances. The challenge is how this subtle therapy, echoing all those subtle energies which together form the universe, will make its voice heard against the cacophony of strident voices out there trying to shout it down as peripheral. Against such vociferous disdain and deep ignorance of what acupuncture can do, I like to range all those satisfied voices of my own and others' patients who in their quiet way bear profound testimony to what I have written here. When I get dispirited by the weight of what is ranged against acupuncture, I comfort myself by thinking of the many future patients to whom we will be able to offer such profound healing. I believe their voices in their thousands and hundreds of thousands, quiet as each may be, will act as a counterweight on acupuncture's side.

A cry from the heart

What follows is a cry from the heart and a cry for the heart, for it is that deepest part of us for which this book is written and which is so often ignored. We have to learn to replace soul within body if we are truly to heal the myriad ills which surround us, and which drag so many people down into chasms of ill-health from which the medical tools generally available often can do little to rescue them. Thus this last section of my book is a form of summons to arms on behalf of the soul, and necessarily includes an indictment of so much that I see as wrong in our modern approach to health. I speak unashamedly with an agenda in mind, and this whole book feeds this agenda. I want as many people as possible to pause in their unquestioning acceptance of received medical opinion and dare to submit it to inspection. I offer what can be seen as an alternative, and one which readers, too, must question, but the blind acceptance of a medical perspective which so blatantly disregards that profoundest part of us is something I regard as deeply disturbing, for it runs counter to the human need and duty to query all things. I hope some part of what I write here raises real questions where before there might have been none.

So what do I see as the modern medical context within which acupuncture must find its place? It is clear to me that anyone concerned with the enhancement of human health and balance must be disturbed by the sheer volume of illnesses we see around us. It can even be said, as it certainly was not when I was young, that the medical scene has shifted from ill-health as being the exception to ill-health as being almost the rule, so frequent are our visits to our doctors. Whence has come such an over-emphasis on the need for outside intervention in our health?

From the perspective of a philosophy of medicine, which, as a matter of course, encompasses within its understanding of health the much profounder concept of soul, Western medicine, for all its apparent sophistication, appears remarkably primitive. Its apparent failure to stem the rising tide of sick bodies flooding its hospitals demands, perhaps, something more than merely additional funding or staff. It is, surely, appropriate for us to question whether the vast resources now pouring into the medical networks are achieving the increase in health such a high percentage of a country's total income warrants. Is such an approach indeed proportionate to the advantages it hopes to confer? Is the population healthier now than it was before such resources were dedicated to restoring or maintaining its health? Are there perhaps cheaper, and indeed more effective, ways of achieving health? And here, of course, I must declare my own vested interest, for acupuncture, so successful in treating the widest range of all human imbalances, both of body and soul, and at so infinitely small a cost compared with its Western counterpart, sits here in the wings, awaiting its turn to take centre stage, if only society were prepared to give it its cue.

It is clear that the advent of a scientific age has meant that science's tentacles have stretched far into medicine, for science is concerned with fathoming the world of matter and has learnt to invent ever more complex instruments to do so, enabling it to probe within us, subjecting every part of us to intense scrutiny. It could be said that it has brought to medicine the worship of detail, turning Western medicine to a great extent into a science of parts. Our bodies, like the hospitals which service them, are cut up and compartmentalized. And this has been done by delving ever deeper within the human body in an attempt to force from it its secrets. In the early days, only the dead body, as corpse and skeleton, was accessible to such probing, but as scientific methods have become more refined and instruments more delicate, a new range of techniques has enabled us to penetrate within the living body itself, whose deepest secrets now lie revealed, and have become subject to increasingly intricate investigations, as each tiny part of us is in turn exposed to X-ray and scan, and probed with scalpel and laser. It is now a common procedure to remove from the body samples of living tissue for detailed analysis by laboratory instruments. No part of us, from our intricate brain to the tiniest nerve, is exempt from such intimate examination.

All such medical procedures sacrifice a sense of the body's unity in their search for the tiniest component dwelling within the smallest cell, and thus tend to demolish its awesome coherence. And as a consequence of such processes of fragmentation, the hospital has become as though a repair shop, to which the human body in distress is despatched in parts, its heart to the cardiology department, its kidneys to the renal department, its nerves to the neurology department. The more a human body comes to be regarded in this way as separate parts rather than as a whole, the more closely it becomes equated with an inanimate object, making it more difficult for us to maintain a dividing line between that which is alive and that which is not. And from there it is but a short step to an assumption that the same investigative approaches which science directs at stick and stone must be sufficient to determine the causes of human ill-health and effect their cure. A concept of health relying predominantly upon physical instruments in this way assumes that the answer to illness must lie in the laboratory. And the hospital, which encloses us with our fellow sick within a building dedicated to the physical relief of suffering, is the inevitable outcome of such a concept.

Great monuments to the supremacy of the body's importance to health, our hospitals are now erected where once temples and cathedrals soared as monuments to the supremacy of the soul. Indeed, some of us would argue that better healing would take place, whatever the god or higher being or force of nature we believe in, if acts of physical healing were carried out in places of spiritual healing and repose. Perhaps those who built sanatoria for the sick in the high mountains in the last century knew something we have forgotten. Lacking penicillin to cure tuberculosis, they transported their patients to the purity of the mountain air in an acknowledgement of nature's powers, if not always to heal, then to give relief.

Perhaps to lie on a balcony looking at the high snowy pastures and breathing in clear mountain air was a better, and certainly a cheaper, way of trying to arrest deterioration than lying enclosed in a hospital room without access to anything but reprocessed air which has passed through the lungs of countless other sick people, often, too, with those faint echoes of nature, the bowl of cut flowers, banished from the bedside for fear of infection. The hospital, sadly, is the antithesis of a place which acknowledges that oneness of all things, for it detaches its patients from their loved ones, places them in cold, impersonal rooms, surrounded by cold, impersonal and often frightening instruments of healing, and ministers only to that part of them, the body which its instruments of investigation detect, ignoring those other parts of the patient which help that body cope, survive, love, hate, write music and great novels, think deep thoughts, and rise above the very miseries which confinement in a hospital often appear to engender rather than to cure.

My voyage away from the world of the physical, the concrete, into a world in which my body has become a shimmering mass of energy, sensitive to the slightest influence, absorbing from all the energies swirling around outside it what it needs to blossom and grow, or to wither and die, has made me ask myself whether this scientific mind of ours, so intent upon foraging among the remains of the body, should not rather draw back the lens of its microscopic eye and allow those tiny parts of us, now so unhappily separated, to rejoin their fellows and replace themselves once more within a larger context. We must beware of following science down that treacherous road which has led to our dismemberment, for, dissected into ever smaller parts, our instruments growing more intricate as the bits of us they try to encompass shrink, we are in danger of becoming mere ruins from which we have drained the very life-blood of our soul.

To one practising a form of medicine which approaches a person as a delicately balanced organism whose health depends upon sensitive adjustments to the stresses of life, as I do, the idea of voluntarily subjecting this delicate mechanism to the brutalities of some forms of modern medical therapy is alien and distressing, and worst of all often unnecessary. But who, faced with the massed ranks of drug companies and equipment manufacturers and medical staff, all reared in a belief that such forms of treatment represent the only way forward, dares to question these procedures except, perhaps, somebody like me, steeped in a completely different medical tradition offering a radically different approach?

Against such a background of demolition, where the elements of the body gradually assume greater importance than the whole from which they have been taken, it is increasingly difficult to maintain any concept of this body as a beautifully balanced unity, however sincere the intention so to do. The practice of medicine has become, doubtless despite itself, a non-holistic practice. It has come to treat the ear, the back, the toe, the throat, the stomach-ache, the migraine, in isolation, with little reference to connections between them. The human body lies in parts before us, as though that slide of a cell magnified by the microscope has its own isolated identity. We take ourselves out of context, thereby running the risk of losing sight of the framework into which all fits. It is as though science, by bowing to the breakdown of the universe, has bowed, too, to the breakdown of Man.

Over the past few centuries or so, abetted by our homage to the gods of science who demand of us allegiance to what is said, often mistakenly, to be provable, the West has appeared to work slowly outwards from a worship of the spirit within us, which dominated previous centuries, to a worship of that spirit's casing, the body. We have felt that if things cannot be reduced to something we can measure, their very existence must be in doubt. We often appear to discard as primitive any beliefs which question whether the findings of science truly reflect the reality of all that is. And thus it is upon the outward manifestation of our being, this body of ours, visible and palpable testimony to our existence, that we understandably concentrate so much of our attention, for is this not within the reassuring compass of our instruments? Perhaps it is that, in a world troubling in its insecurity, the apparent solidity of the physical reassures us, and upon this comfort we have learnt to rely, for things we can touch and see appear safe. The body feels so solid, so reassuringly there. Of this, we comfort ourselves, there can be no doubt.

It is one of the deficiencies of Western medicine that it has shown no interest in exploring the concept of a soul within our body, and presupposes a body like some cardboard cut-out, which can be manipulated and moved around as though a discrete, detached entity, a thing standing alone. And for such an object – for as an object it truly is regarded – what need do we have to be concerned about what we do to it and where we do those things? Hence the appalling disregard for the indignities to which we subject our body in the name of restoring health, the incisions, the instruments prodded down, up and into every bit of us, the drugs flooding our arteries with toxic substances. A physician friend of mine told me recently that he often finds that the procedures he asks his patients to undergo to assess whether they are ill are worse than the illnesses themselves for which they are being tested.

Indeed, viewed at its simplest level, can something that makes you feel worse really get you better? Many of Western medicine's attempts at healing intrude, disturb, cause pain and distress, and some leave us worse off than we were before. How many are saved or are made worse by such interventions? Is it possible that many are made more sick for the sake of the few who get well? All these are valid questions to be asked. An industry, which is what much Western medicine now is, driven by market forces which include telling the state, its paymaster, how many procedures or how many new drugs it needs, and how much new equipment it needs, has no incentive to query the rationale for all this increased expenditure, for to do this is to query its very raison d'être.

And we show as little regard for the environment in which all these terrifying interventions take place, the frightening machines, the lack of natural air, even the ban on plants and flowers in the hospital wards of the most sick, as if such harmless, natural and beautiful things bring with them a greater chance of disease than dealing with the high incidence of hospital-induced infections. The cold and sterile impersonality of it all! A patient often confronting alone a machine, or even, oh horror, left alone inside a machine, the helpers ducking for safety out of sight behind a screen, protecting themselves from the deadly rays they expose their patients to. What must this do to our body's defences, that precious immune system attempting to shield us from attack? How many people ask such questions? Or query whether there may be more effective ways of treating such illnesses?

A patient of mine under hospital treatment for a hyperactive thyroid was witness to the extraordinary pass to which health care has now come. She was told by her specialist that he needed to check her thyroid function by injecting into it radioactive iodine and monitoring its progress over time. When she protested that she did not wish to undergo such a procedure, she was told that, although her specialist, too, did not regard the test as absolutely essential, 'I have all this equipment here I am supposed to use'. A doctor friend told me recently of a hospital basement stocked with unused state-of-the-art equipment for which the hospital had neither the staff, the funds nor the need, and about whose benefits they were unclear, but which they had to order 'otherwise all our research funding will dry up'. This is a world of healing gone mad.

The medicalized society

Western medicine, by concentrating on the outside of things, has also encouraged us to use external means to repulse and vanquish what it regards as the attacks upon the body we call by the name of illnesses, turning them into something alien and apart, things forcefully to be removed or obliterated, rather than unhappy but still organically connected parts of the whole. And the step from here to considering the body as a thing out there, and hence always a possible foe to be vanquished, is only too easily taken. We have devised many ways of attacking what we regard as these invaders of the body, handing our health over to others as we allow our bodies to be cut open, prodded and dissected, and as we take our many drugs, as though in each artificially produced pill lies the secret to all health.

Then, too, the very real achievements of science which have yielded obvious benefits, such as the invention of antibiotics or hip replacements and all manner of ways of keeping us alive where before we would have died, have altered our mindset. Success in one area has led us to press for medical successes wider afield. If we don't now have to fall sick with tuberculosis or smallpox, or die of septicaemia (although here, too, the over-prescription of antibiotics has wreaked its own havoc), then perhaps we should protest when we have any kind of pain which cannot be alleviated, and demand, as we increasingly do, that something be done, even if the doing of this something may in the end prove fruitless. All this pressure to act rather than to wait or to suffer has made us far less prepared to tolerate discomfort, however temporary and however minor. We demand action from our doctors to whom we turn ever more frequently as soon as we experience the slightest twinge. And because they in turn work within a system which assumes that medicine is always there to act rather than to encourage us to wait or suffer, when they themselves feel unable to do something they pass us on to others, whose more specialized skills they think must surely be able to succeed where they have failed.

GPs' surgeries often tend, therefore, to be the first rather than the last stopping-point in our search for health, for so worried are doctors that they may be accused of overlooking some serious illness that they only too easily play on our fears by passing our files over to one or other hospital department, as though seeking to absolve themselves of responsibility. It is rare for us to be told to wait a little longer or to be offered the soothing words or sugary placebos of former years which might have sent many of us away surprisingly happier for having been offered something, anything. And often, perhaps, that is all that may be needed, for time, surprisingly often, cures. The problem, though, is that it doesn't do this in all cases, far from it, and the spectre of an undetected serious pathological condition haunts all that Western medicine does, so that the fear this engenders has skewed the whole of our medical system in the direction of intervention in case something life-threatening has been overlooked. This means that even a slightly pathological state receives the same drastic attention as the most serious condition. And all drastic procedures have their risk.

Once in hospital hands, we often find they never let us go, for one test or another, imperfect as all tests must be, may surprisingly often yield a slightly ambiguous result which demands a different test or a further check-up later on, leaving us forever waiting for what we anticipate may be a dreaded result, as though shackled to a permanent pathological prognosis. This is a depressingly frequent occurrence, for no doctor appears to dare sign us off for fear of future repercussions.

What we now have is what I call a medicalized society where we are so worried that we might fail to detect a serious illness in time that we spend a lifetime of often good health worrying ourselves sick by testing for it. Recently, a young patient of mine who is coming to the end of her pregnancy told me that there had not been a single day of this pregnancy, an event which she greeted with great joy, when she was not frightened of the result of some test or other she was encouraged to undergo with little understanding of its need and even less of the repercussions on her of its results. And even preparing for the birth has now become a time of some confusion where birth plans, almost invariably thrown out by the ever-differing realities of the birth itself, have to be drawn up with little understanding of what the complexities of any birth demand. It appears that the more we think we know about the physical functioning of the different parts of our body, the greater the danger that this knowledge can lead us away from the natural and the healthy into a world where the unnatural, the unbalanced, the us-as-ill-or-about-to-be-ill-people, rules.

All this leads to the expectation that we have a right not to be ill and an equal right to demand that somebody, something, out there puts things right for us, and hence that we are justified in our often frantic search for cures. And yet in all this medicalization of life we have given little thought so far to what procedures and interventions are appropriate for which age or for which stage of an illness, and for the risks inherent in any of these procedures, so that an 80-year-old may be offered surgery which those prescribing it know may well do little to enhance quality of life, and in many cases may be distressing in itself, and a terminally ill patient may be offered treatments which do nothing but prolong a pain-ridden life. Nor do many people question whether it is appropriate, or ultimately healthy, for a 55-year-old woman, a patient of mine, to be encouraged to continue to take hormone replacement therapy which leads her to haemorrhage quite badly every month with inappropriate periods which should have run their natural course years ago. And she has had to be put on further medication for the anaemia this has caused, in effect being prescribed a further medication to undo the damage done by the original medication. How necessary, too, is much drastic surgery, and how carefully monitored are the prescriptions of radio- or chemotherapy, all procedures which in themselves are known to be harmful, however benign the intent of those prescribing them? These are all valid questions, not to be shirked because their implications may be disturbing.

In this climate, where we have lost a balanced perspective on our health, the natural processes of growing old and dying also now evoke increasing fear for appearing unnatural, stoked by a culture built upon the illusion that old age and death should somehow not be our fate (witness, here, the facelifts, the body suctioning, the slimming cures, the gyms, all efforts to stem a remorseless tide) that we have allowed a whole medical industry to grow up which fosters this illusion, and fights to the death any attempt to question the validity of what it does. And because we have a natural fear of growing ill, and are now often ill-prepared to contemplate our own death, anything which appears to soothe these fears will be welcome, however illusory what is offered. In fact, the more illusory the goods on offer (eternal youth, endless health), the more they buy into this need of ours to hide from reality, and the more readily we accept them.

If a hospital, with its myriad of tests and procedures, can convince us that the sheer number of these interventions adds to our chances of regaining health, then we will devise more and more tests to fill this need, shouting down anybody who dares question whether they actually yield anything other than distress, let alone lead to greater health. The medical edifice we have built up is so huge and all-powerful, has its own imperatives and is so self-perpetuating, that if one drug or intervention or test fails and damages us, another is immediately asked for. Few query whether it is always by such brutal invasive procedures that the delicate balance of our health can be restored.

What if the attempt at a cure is worse than the illness itself? Who is there prepared to evaluate this, or even to query? Who is there to collect evidence on the effectiveness of different forms of drug therapy, or the mastectomies and hysterectomies, so haphazardly and often needlessly carried out? Instead, the vast juggernaut rolls on, no doubt helping many, but, in its inexorable advance, damaging many, too. And who would dare question in this way? Would not such a person be accused of denying patients their right to health? In all the current discussions about the cost of healthcare, the absence of any radical public questioning of the need to increase expenditure is depressingly noticeable. There appears to be little incentive to examine whether increased expenditure leads to increased health. And so far much of the resources poured into the national health service here in Britain have manifestly not led to better health, else our hospitals would be emptying. The scale of illnesses we are faced with has certainly not diminished, however massive the weapons we have arrayed against them. And, to our dismay, we have found that these weapons bring with them their own deadly problems. Surely the vast resources we devote to health matters would have proved sufficient by now, if not to eliminate, at least to reduce to manageable proportions, the scale of illness which confronts us. Whence then the long and ever longer queues for hospital beds?

One of the many areas to be re-assessed, too, is the Western reliance on statistics. The trouble with statistics is that they are illusory. They appear to be based on scientific fact, and offer scientific validity, but they have no meaning whatsoever in the individual case. If a test is said to offer a 60% probability of establishing that a person is likely to suffer a heart-attack, am I in the 60% category of the sick or in the 40% category of the well? No-one can tell me this, but human nature being as it is, all 100% of us are unlikely to sleep easily at night with such a statistic hovering over our heads. And yet we may never fall ill. What a way to approach health, and what an indictment of a system that condemns both the sick and the well to such frightening uncertainty. We know that fears of this kind which hover over much of Western medicine must affect our ability to remain healthy, for the most damaging thing is for us to lose hope, to become dispirited and give up. And therein lies deep danger, for there is no more effective defence against illness than our own deep belief that we have the ability to regain health. Attack this belief by the corrosive pessimism inherent in the whole Western medicine system, and you undermine the whole structure of health.

The current approach to health has become such a no-go area that it requires much bravery to query whether this approach is the correct one. Recently a leading cancer specialist was hounded by the press for daring to question the safety and usefulness of carrying out so many mammograms. These are questions we often shrink from asking, particularly because any questioning of current medical practice causes distress to those at the moment undergoing the various forms of treatment it prescribes. Merely to ask, as has recently been done publicly, whether the use of radiotherapy in treating breast cancer is a safe procedure, has caused one of my patients, herself receiving this treatment, to feel as though her last hope had been taken from her.

The implications for our health of such taboos are frightening. But if we care about our health and our children's future, this is terrain we must venture upon, however risky the undertaking, and however strongly this appears to fly in the face of accepted assumptions. And here again we face the difficulty presented by the sheer size of the task facing us. The sick are rarely fit persons to evaluate the treatment they are receiving, and most are actively discouraged from enquiring too deeply as to the chances of success and rates of failure. This task must fall to those not themselves involved in the treatment, either as practitioners or patients.

How can an individual gain sufficient information about the complexities of modern therapeutic procedures, when even those prescribing such treatments are often not in a position to evaluate them properly, depending for much of their knowledge upon results of drug trials carried out by drug companies with very vested interests, and upon what little research has been done? In this respect, I found it highly disturbing to read recently how little was apparently known even now about acceptable drug dosages for children.

Gravely ill patients will usually prefer to be offered something on to which to pin their hopes, however unpleasant and distressing its effects. Indeed, there is often a belief that the very unpleasantness of the treatment acts in some way as an appropriate and necessary counterweight to the unpleasantness of the illness, on the age-old principle of 'if it's nasty, it must be doing me some good'. I often feel that in future times the mere hundred years or so when Western medicine has dominated the world of health, as it does now, may come to be regarded in some areas, such as those relating to excessive intervention by drug and surgery, as a barbaric age, the height of man's tampering futilely and often fatally with nature. It may well be that in future centuries, when the true value of such treatments has been properly assessed, some of these radical, invasive treatments will be regarded as belonging to one of the dark ages of medicine. We need only read the newspaper headlines, too, as the risks involved in producing one drug after another are highlighted to see how far we have gone down the road of almost institutionalized acceptance of the medical industry's interference in our health. We hand ourselves over often unquestioningly, no longer insisting on being masters of our fate.

It could be argued that the methods by which modern Western medicine at present attempts to restore our bodies to health appear to gain increased importance the more they distance themselves from whatever the natural world can provide. Here we can call as witness once more the vast hospital networks in which the ill are offered help from an array of man-made instruments and man-made medicines in surroundings as far removed from the natural as can be imagined, and in which the only natural things to be found, apart perhaps from the odd potted plant or bunch of flowers, even if these are allowed, are the human beings they house. Even the air these inmates breathe has to be recycled, for now no modern hospital window is allowed to open on to the outside world. Medical equipment has the effect of severing us from nature, not only isolating the body, and increasingly isolating the parts within the body, one from the other, but of isolating the individual sick person not only from his family and the well, but from the very air he breathes and the ground beneath his feet. We place a patient in hospital as though in solitary confinement.

Taken together with the intricate admission procedures, security checks and locks, this has become a healing world as though deliberately sealing itself from the outside, cutting patients off from their natural habitat. Natural protection having been regarded as having failed, the sick are handed over to the man-made. And nature, once turned thus into our enemy, has a habit of revenging itself. And this is where I like to think acupuncture finds its true place, for it seeks to harness the natural in its attempt to redress imbalance and disease, using our patients' own energies to do so.

When I was first a student, I was delighted to be told that I should start to see myself as an instrument of nature. I found this title at first awesome, but I have since come to wear it with growing pride, for I feel that it assigns me a place as part of the natural forces which I attempt to draw upon to restore my patients to health.

A vision for acupuncture

Sometimes, weighed down by what I often see as the struggle to maintain my own perspective on health against a background dominated by quite a different viewpoint, I give myself a moment of respite by imagining a world of health based upon the principles I have outlined here in relation to acupuncture. And I like to extrapolate these thoughts out to form a vision of a completely different approach to health. This vision would contain within it some of the discoveries of Western medicine but would restrict these to a large extent to those areas of health which deal with acute and extreme cases requiring, perhaps, but not always, immediate, more drastic interventions. Where these two worlds, the world of acupuncture and other forms of what I call natural healing, and the world of Western medicine meet, and how far they can interrelate, is something that requires much greater debate than I can give it here, but what I write below is my first attempt at formulating a different approach which takes account of what acupuncture can offer, and one which I passionately feel can offer many solutions, infinitely more cheaply and less invasively, for the often intractable problems which pour into GPs' surgeries.

But it is a vision which starts from a radically different viewpoint, and predicates a health system whose resources are concentrated, not on equipment, research methodologies and drugs, but on providing patients with a high level of personal support and attention. It is clear that the one-to-one relationship I have with my patients throughout the time of their care with me, multiplied by each patient that I see, compares unfavourably with the few minutes of a GP's or consultant's time, but for a true comparison we have to offset this with the minimum level of additional support I need in terms of my equipment and the staffing of my clinic, if indeed I need any staff apart from myself. My equipment, too, is contained within a small box I can carry in a bag. The savings I can make compared with the much greater expenditure surrounding Western medical procedures could fund an almost limitless number of acupuncturists and other complementary healers.

But how, you may well ask, do I go about treating many of the manifold and differing conditions which flood our hospitals? Surely what I have to offer cannot replace the extensive knowledge of the body and its processes gained by Western medicine, and added to every day by new research? Am I not being arrogant in thinking that I, in my small way, can offer something which can compete with what that vast edifice of accumulated scientific knowledge has to offer? Are the claims I make for acupuncture not too audacious, out of proportion to what it can achieve?

To judge for themselves, I ask my readers to follow me as I treat some of my patients. It may surprise some of those reading these descriptions to discover how wide acupuncture's remit is, so wide, indeed, that it can be compared favourably with its Western counterpart, even when dealing with the most serious illnesses. I will use as examples some patients that came to my practice this week. As before, I have changed names, and altered enough of the details to protect my patients' identities.

My first patient, Josephine, came to me to help her conceive again at 43, having tried unsuccessfully to do so for the previous two years. The extreme tiredness which she had suffered from for months was confirmed by my initial reading of her pulses which showed almost no energy in any of the 12 officials. This indicated a major blockage in the two main sources of energy which feed the five elements, which we call by the name of Governor and Conception Vessels. This can be one of the causes of infertility or menstrual problems, and when corrected happily equally often their solution. She had had an extremely traumatic birth of her second child, and was also beset by all sorts of doubts as to whether her husband wanted another baby, and by unresolved conflicts around her family from her early life, which added many emotional reasons for such a major blocking of energy. This all led to a sense of deep despair within her which made her feel, she admitted, that she was unworthy to have another child. It could be said that she closed herself down. She has responded well to a mere handful of treatments, and is now very happily pregnant, and came this week for her monthly check-up treatment to ensure that all is well. Her element is Fire, and strengthening this element is enabling her to reaffirm her sense of joy in her life, giving herself the warmth to allow her to nourish another little soul.

I have had many similar patients, each despairing of conceiving or with a history of miscarriages, one of whom had a child at the age of 47, conceived, she herself insists, because of a spring treatment I gave her. She came for what we call a seasonal treatment one spring, long after abandoning all hope of having a baby, and perhaps indeed it was the boost to her Wood element, with its push towards the creation of new life, which gave her energy what it needed. We will never know, but she is sure it was the treatment which did the trick.

Another patient this week is a young man who suffers from very violent mood swings which frighten him by their intensity and he is worried that he may harm his girlfriend in one of his uncontrollable bouts of anger. He has been under different forms of psychiatric care for some time and just managed to struggle through university without breaking down. Now that he is out in the world, his fears, held a little in check by the close relationships he formed at university, have surfaced again and he feels his fragile control slipping. A very repressive family life, with high-achieving parents and an older sibling who could do no wrong in their eyes, have, I am sure, played a part in unbalancing him so that he is finding it increasingly difficult to leave home to go to work. After our first encounter last week, I felt it was the Metal element which is crumbling under the stress, Metal's cutting anger when it finds itself inadequate revealing itself in the phantasies of violence which he is unable to escape from. Again, I have every hope that strengthening the Metal element, and thus increasing his sense of self-worth, will remove some of the overpowering feelings of inadequacy which fuel his anger. My experience of similar situations in other patients leads me to feel confident that I can help him regain control, and he tells me that the few treatments he has had have already made him feel that he is less prey to his emotions.

At least seven more of the patients I have treated this week can be said to be coming for help with emotional problems. Most, but not all, originally came with physical complaints, and are continuing their treatment once these have improved, but at wider intervals, because of the emotional balance they feel acupuncture offers them. The physical complaints ranged from irritable bowel syndrome, severe back-ache, tendonitis, irregular periods, headaches to arthritis, all these conditions now either no longer there or so fleetingly there that my patients no longer mention them as the reason for coming for treatment.

Two more of my patients have much more serious complaints, one lung cancer and the other breast cancer. One patient is undergoing chemotherapy at the moment and the other now visits the hospital only for her six-monthly check-ups. Both patients would be considered as being or having been severely ill. The acupuncture treatment for the patient having chemotherapy helps him maintain his blood levels at a sufficiently high level to make it possible for him to have his chemotherapy treatments, and prevents much of the resultant nausea. The other patient, in remission now for ten years, is here for maintenance treatment. In both patients treatment reinforces the elements' power to support their immune system in its work of holding the cancers at bay and will, we all hope, muster sufficient defences to fight any further attack upon them.

I have had many cancer patients who have successfully fended off a recurrence of their illnesses, whether due to acupuncture or not I cannot confirm, since all had conventional medical treatment as well, but in sufficient numbers and with sufficient indications from the comments of their Western medical teams to suggest that acupuncture has played an integral role in their improvement. Each acupuncture treatment allows the different energies to flow with greater strength around body and soul, and will thus, I hope, in these two patients of mine, also prevent any future breakdowns such as have occurred before.

Acupuncture treatment here is not so much an attack upon the body, as with Western procedures which treat cancers as invaders to be defeated, but as a way of mobilizing the body's own defence systems in an attempt to reintegrate a diseased part of the body back into its healthier surroundings. One of today's patients told me that the specialist had said that the tumour in his lung had reduced in size and those in his bones 'appeared to be integrating themselves more fully, strengthening the bone structures'. He is also having some experimental drug therapy and no doubt his specialist will ascribe his improvement to this, and who is to say he is not right? And yet, having observed how he improved well before starting this new drug regime, he and I are confident that acupuncture has played an important part in his continuing recovery.

Turning now to the less seriously ill of this week's patients, three fall into the category which GPs might call non-specific illnesses, with no obvious physical symptoms except those of tiredness, sleeplessness or mild discomfort. It is this category of patient with which acupuncture has such a high success rate, for it is precisely those early signs of not feeling well which indicate the start of imbalances in the elements which a few treatments are likely to set right. I like to dwell on the number of such patients whose treatment has enabled them to ward off the onset of more serious conditions later. By correcting such imbalances at a sufficiently early stage, the tiny adjustments to unbalanced energy which the needle makes can prevent the major imbalances which require more urgent interventions later on.

And finally I have treated four patients this week who come only occasionally now, the first every 6 months and the other three every 2–4 months, each of them regarding their treatment as a form of preventive therapy. They now have no obvious physical symptoms, although all had originally some physical complaints which both they and I have now forgotten about, so long ago were their first treatments and so successfully were these conditions eliminated. They all tell me that acupuncture keeps them balanced both physically and emotionally, and if anything it is much more for their emotional equilibrium that they now say they continue treatment. In each case, the strengthening of their particular element in whatever way I feel is appropriate for them on this particular day sends them away again in good health and good heart for a further few months.

CHAPTER 11

Closing the Circle

In endeavouring to fashion for myself some understanding of the nature of human individuality as expressed within the elements, I have come to my own vision of the human dilemma with which I will conclude this book. I would ask you to read this as my homage to the awesome depths within each of us and to the potential each of us has to find within these depths that pure jewel at the heart of us which is our understanding and acceptance of who we are. What I write here is my personal attempt to make sense of the profound nature of the human being, but it is no more speculative, I venture to say, than any of the many constantly changing and disputed theories of the origin of all things and the nature of our being. It satisfies my sense of the poetry of life and the rhythms of things.

And it is fitting that it is upon the Water element, that most mysterious source of all life, that I call to draw this book to a close, as it draws a circle round all that is. Like a constant and distant sea murmur, tempting us with its nostalgic memories of a long-forgotten, long-desired time when we were at one with all that is, Water gently sings us its siren songs of peace. For a brief and well-deserved while, the world rests from its labours, lulled to sleep in its soft arms. The great circle of life drawn around the universe closes us in its winter sleep, each winter a tiny death, and death itself no more than an extension of our annual dying.

As the waters close over our heads, how tempting it would be to remain floating effortlessly and eternally in this watery womb. Thus must the universe have felt before that first outwards explosion broke the whole into parts, made the complete incomplete. Sufficient unto itself, its own beginning and end, it would have had no need of anything beyond itself, lazing its life away in peaceful self-contemplation, a dense and tight ball rolling endlessly through time. Surely, we ask ourselves, this must be all that we seek, the infinite comfort of staying forever as we are, unchallenged and complete, our days unnumbered, our gaze fixed on infinity, desireless, indivisible, in glorious and satisfied peace.

And yet the universe, offered this great gift of unity, chose instead to tear itself into fragments. And therein lies the wonder, for the whole of creation chose the difficult path. It sacrificed the peace and harmony of its original unity for the strife and confusion of disunity, for when it was one, all it could be was itself, but when it became many, manifold, too, became its desires. What immense and awe-inspiring purpose could possibly justify such a courageous act of self-destruction? Perhaps, who knows, that great hand holding all in its grasp may have grown momentarily tired of its own self-absorption and slackened its hold. And the world, awaiting only such a moment to take its chance, escaped through its half-opened fingers. There may be a time in the future when this great hand decides to take a rest from its present labours and draw back to its still centre (and astronomers predict this), but now is not that time. Restlessly dividing and combining, flying apart and fusing together, the universe seethes with creative activity, in which, like it or not, we are forced to take part. As the great circle broke apart, the challenge of change crept in, to tantalize and tempt and dissatisfy, like some eternal itch in the side of the universe, and into the pattern of things slipped the yearning for what each has not got, for all things must henceforth feel themselves incomplete.

We, too, are born incomplete, torn before time from the womb, defenceless, unable to sustain ourselves alone, struggling to comprehend for what purpose we should thus have been abandoned, and given a mere handspan of years in which to make something of this great puzzle. In slipping each into our solitary life, we have detached ourselves from the great cosmic embrace to stand solitary and alone. What a price we could be said to pay for the right to an individual life. We could feel lost, our life a mere breath drawn at the whim of some arbitrary and indifferent god, our presence on this small, dark planet spinning in vast space an event of total meaninglessness. We could seem to be scratching for significance upon the surface of our life, like a hen pecking at the dust.

Little wonder that many of us, faced by such a gigantic and daunting task, choose rather to bury our heads in incuriosity, and shut our eyes tight to the awesome spaces surrounding us. But those with the courage to open their eyes wide will find themselves rewarded by visions of such beauty as to make a mockery of their doubts. For the view of all things revealed to our wondering gaze as we complete our journey around the elements must fill us with hushed awe. That giant hand holding all in its grasp, as it hovers over the universe, pointing here, directing there, changing the course of the years, calling life into existence, decreeing its death, has not, in its endless and exacting work, forgotten us. On each of our heads it lays a hand of blessing. Mine it has blessed with its finger of Fire, and has thereby given me meaning.

Just as those constellations pursuing their sweeping course through infinite space in their passing place upon the brow of each of us the mark of our birth-time, branding one of us Aries, another Taurus, so, too, the elements pause for a slight moment in their endless wheeling to stamp their individual signatures upon us. As the wheel of the elements turns endlessly from beginning to end, from birth to death, a tiny hesitation, the slightest opening, appears in its smooth flow, allowing just sufficient space for us to slip in at our birth and join the flow of life. And there where we are marked with that stamp of our individuality there remains forever a slight wound, an opening to the great universe beyond. It is our loophole to the infinite, a place through which we can grow or shrink.

And the point at which we flow into the circle remains for us forever an imperfection, a tender umbilicus still aching from that first brutal cut which severed us from the whole and propelled us, reluctantly, into our own separate identity. Thus we are given our individual yearning, each our own dissatisfaction, with which we will struggle throughout our life. For each of us this struggle takes place before the gate of one of our guardian elements, for it is there that the forces of change are encamped and their attention concentrated. One element stands for a lifetime at our shoulder, a guardian of what we do, and when we ignore its warning signs of distress, we will fall ill, whether in body or soul. Its sheltering hand placed over us is thus a guide, a wayfinder. It signals the direction in which we must pursue our life.

And it can direct us outwards from the centre to any of the four points of the compass, pointing us for a lifetime in one of five directions. Those of us blessed with Wood's green finger will head east towards the rising sun, the spring of the year, the bud on the tree and hope. Those of us branded by Fire will turn our faces longingly towards the south, the noonday sun, the great joys of summer and love. Metal's cooler hand upon us turns us towards the west, the dying of the light, and grief for all those things we have to lose, and the flowing hands of Water bear us north, and dip us down, deep down into the dark and fearsome depths of our winter sleep. And towards the centre from which all radiates outwards, back towards the very axis of this inner world of energy, are drawn those of us destined to live our lives enfolded within Earth's arms. Our time, then, will be the time of harvest, that great turning-point of the year, when the earth draws back down to itself all that has borne fruit upon its surface, and the year slowly tilts from yang to yin.

And we must remain with our eyes fixed firmly eastwards if Wood has blessed us, or northwards if Water has been chosen as our home. This will be the direction of our fulfilment, however much we may yearn to turn our steps elsewhere. In this direction only lies our growth. It will thus be our destiny always to be ourselves, always to yearn for the comforts of Earth or ache with the regrets of Metal, to crave the strong structure of Wood or the smiling happinesses of Fire, and to need forever Water's reassurance that it will survive.

All these longings we will have in some proportion, for life is the energies of all the five elements flowing as a stream through us, but our guardian element will give our life its dominant colour and texture, and that one longing which this element places closest to our heart will dictate the shape of our life. To satisfy it must be our aim. All illness then is a stumbling sideways into the undergrowth, a turning aside from the clear path of our true self along which our guardian element points us. We pursue for a lifetime each our own complicated and individual destiny. And that destiny is closely related to the burdens and delights, hopes and despairs our guardian element bestows upon us as gifts for life. It is the means by which that cosmic purpose works itself out at the human level, for the great forces of the cosmos, scattering wide the universe, still retain a tight hold on all so dispersed. The universe speaks through each of us, and those few moments when we emerge briefly and triumphantly as ourselves give us meaning.

The opening in the great circle of energy through which we slip into life will remain to challenge and excite us, beckoning us to venture out beyond ourselves. But, oh, the temptation to stay as we are, to cower back down and tuck ourselves firmly away within the safety of the familiar. How simple it would be to turn our backs on those glimpses of change, and deny ourselves development. But when our guardian element puts its mark upon us and places us for our lifetime under its protection it expects something in return for its patronage, for no gift is given us to squander. We have the lifelong responsibility of using it wisely.

In some profound way there lies a paradox at the heart of each one of us. It is almost as though that for which we long the most is denied us, our guardian element pointing the way forward to our fulfilment and yet in some way denying us what we most ardently seek, for there where that blessing has branded us, there will remain forever a wound to remind us, like Achilles his heel, that we are imperfect and vulnerable. And that very imperfection is our gift, for our yearning to become whole again will drive us onwards, all things seeking their own way back to that original unity of which they retain a memory. Perhaps, then, we are necessarily incomplete. How better to encourage development and growth than by denying us our wholeness and making us yearn for what we no longer have, for then our very incompletion acts as our spur? And to the hands of our guardian element is entrusted the task of issuing that denial. Nurturing and supporting, protecting and encouraging, yet it withholds its most precious gift, the bestowal of all it knows, aware, as all good teachers are, that the only true learning is by deprivation and disappointment. Lazy as we are, we learn not by our pleasures, for these only lull us into inactivity, but by our pains, and who knows better than our guardian what these are?

And thus it is at this point where the elements open their arms to welcome us that we confront that most audacious and demanding of tasks of turning a circle into a spiral.

Printed in Great
Britain
by Amazon